SABRINA DE FEDERICIS

Choose to TREAT the allergy, not to numb the symptoms

NO MORE TISSUES

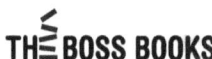

Dedicated to my son Simone and to all those with allergies who want to breathe again

NO MORE TISSUES
Sabrina de Federicis

Design by The Boss Books Editions

One Hour Marketing Srl
via Torino 9, 21013 Gallarate (VA)
www.libridimpresa.it

www.thebossbooks.com

THE BOSS BOOKS

Copyright © 2024 Sabrina de Federicis
All rights reserved.
This book or parts thereof may not be reproduced or transmitted in any form by any means—electronic, mechanical, photocopy, recording, or otherwise—without prior written permission of the Author.

ISBN 9791281915107

TABLE OF CONTENTS

Preface	9
Preamble	13
Chapter 1 – A planet of allergic people	**19**
The therapy that exists (but that only few know about)	22
The "everything and now"	26
The National Health System is also responsible	28
Is it a vaccine?	29
The origins	30
Allergies are not to be underestimated	31
The time factor	34
Who I am	36
A palaeontologist on loan to the pharmaceutical industry	36

TABLE OF CONTENTS

Chapter 2 – Case history: the plane, the pilot and the cat — 41

Chapter 3 – Case history: the lawyer and the lichwort — 53

Chapter 4 – Case history: him, her and the cats — 63

Chapter 5 – Case history: obstacle jumping — 71

Chapter 6 – Case history: the underwater lawyer — 81

Chapter 7 – Case history: companion snails — 89

Chapter 8 – The desensitization therapy — 99

Chapter 9 – The nhs and the desensitization therapies: who pays for them? Cost or value? — 119

Chapter 10 – What if the little prince had been allergic? — 127

TABLE OF CONTENTS

Conclusions	133
Glossary	139
Afterword by Paolo Ciani	143
Afterword by Gianfranco Fortunato	149
Thank you for reading this far!	153
Acknowledgements	157
Biography	161
Appendix	162

> Take good care of your body, it's the only place you have to live.

Jim Rohn

PREFACE

Examples are the best way to learn.

I am delighted to write this new preface for the second edition of *No More Tissues*, especially because the two years since its first publication invite us to reflect. What has occurred during this time, from various perspectives, is extraordinary. The wide circulation of this book has significantly contributed to raising awareness about allergies. Its simple structure and engaging stories allow readers to explore common scenarios faced by allergy sufferers through real-life episodes, presented with a touch of humor. Seneca, the great Roman philosopher, once said, *"The path to learning is long if you go by rules, but short and effective if you proceed by examples"*. It is precisely this idea that inspired Sabrina to write this book in a straightforward and relatable style.

Allergies should not be underestimated. Sneezing a few times in spring or occasionally blowing your nose might seem trivial, but such issues can have serious consequences on the quality of life of those affected, often leading them to withdraw socially.

Consider those who are allergic to certain plants and avoid

countryside walks for fear of a respiratory crisis. Or those with food allergies who skip restaurant outings to avoid a potentially severe reaction to hidden ingredients. Some are allergic to dust and spend excessive time cleaning their homes, finding it challenging to go anywhere else, including work or school. Others are allergic to pets and not only forgo having one at home but must also avoid visiting friends who do.

Allergies, therefore, are not mere inconveniences; they are conditions that can disrupt the well-being of individuals and those around them, significantly interfering with social relationships and drastically lowering the quality of life.

The figures suggested by epidemiology confirm an ever-increasing spread of allergies in all districts. It's important to note that allergies can manifest in various ways, affecting the nose, eyes, gastrointestinal system, skin, and lungs, often causing symptoms in multiple areas simultaneously.

The solution, though not widely recognized, is the so-called desensitizing therapy; This is the only treatment that can effectively cure allergies and lead to their remission.

An allergist can prescribe a personalized treatment involving the administration of small doses of the allergen itself. This process trains the immune system to recognize the substance as harmless, preventing symptoms upon future exposure. In essence, the goal is to restore the well-being of allergy sufferers.

This book serves as an essential tool for raising public awareness about allergies, a condition often trivialized, and for spreading knowledge about a definitive solution.

If allergies can profoundly alter the lives of those affected and their loved ones, it is equally true that **they can be treated, enabling individuals to return to enjoying life**, nature, and meaningful relationships without the fear of falling ill. The cases shared in this book, though narrated with humour and lightness, are real, and the individuals involved have happily resumed their lives in full health.

Dr. Andrea Di Rienzo Businco
Specialist in Allergology and Clinical Immunology

"The story within the story: two years with *Butta Via i Fazzoletti*.

PREAMBLE

Writing a book is a great emotion, dedicating it to your child is exciting, creating it for a social and informative purpose is, to say the least, electrifying. Two years have passed, 700 days since *Butta Via i Fazzoletti* [No More Tissues - TN] debuted and I still can't believe in how many things have happened in this short period of time. I hoped for interest, curiosity, but I didn't expect such a real awakening of the allergic population and of the political forces themselves, often distracted by internal squabbles and power play. Ten thousand people have downloaded the book in PDF format from the homonymous blog absolutely free of charge. This is because, according to me, disseminating does not mean profiting but making your knowledge and experience available to others. I met so many people during the presentation tour that I almost struggle to believe it.

Allergy sufferers, parents of children living with this problem, distressed grandparents who wanted to know more, friends of allergy sufferers who wanted to delve deeper into the topic: a humankind ready to use its time to listen, ask questions and understand. They all came with openness and enthusiasm despite, at times, the harsh weather conditions and the cold winter nights. Their testimonies have highlighted to me even more the deep detachment between healthcare and people with allergies. Nevertheless, the problem is important. 12 million people in Italy show symptoms related to a respiratory allergy and there is no age groups excluded from this phenomenon. Above all, it confirms the perception of allergy as a "nuisance" and not a real pathology and the habit of "quickly fixing" the problem with the use or abuse of antihistamines and cortisone.

The book and politics

Butta Via i Fazzoletti had the honour, at its debut, of an afterword written by the Lazio regional Councillor, MP Paolo Ciani, now a Demos member of the Chamber of Deputies. Paolo, whom I deeply thank, is a man of rare sensitivity and pragmatism and, according to my opinion, a politician who follows words with concrete facts. During his mandate in the Lazio Region, he promoted a motion so that the region, home to the capital city, would also support - through a joint participation - the citizen's expenditure for the drugs that are the basis of the desensitizing therapy (Name Patients products drugs) recognized by the World Health Organization as the only curative therapy and, unlike Italy, widely used throughout Europe. The motion was presented again in July, as the government of the region had changed: Paolo Ciani did not let the issue drop. Indeed, once elected Member of the Chamber of Deputies, he decided to propose an interparliamentary group, together with Senator Sbrollini, that would shine a spotlight on the little-considered topic of allergies.
The consulted MPs have joined the initiative, together with the university and hospital scientific societies, the patient associations,

PREAMBLE

"Cittadinanza Attiva" and many others. This has created an inclusive working table, to which I was invited to participate precisely in the field of communication, in my role as a scientific communicator, which has produced a legislative pact with 10 points focused on the person with allergies. I like to remember point number 8, in which the importance of the desensitizing therapy and related drugs is underlined, both with AIC and under the NPP label and the obligation of a uniformity of therapeutic availability in all Italian regions, in full compliance with the Constitution and Article 32. Together with MP Ciani of Demos, we share this substantial ethical aspect: quality of health care treatment among all Italian regions. As a matter of facts, we cannot accept such a marked disparity, such as the one that exists today and which finds in the diversity of distribution of the desensitizing therapy among the various regions, only the tip of the iceberg of the problem of an individualism that divides instead of connecting and contributing to the creation of a community. The legislative pact has generated an interpellation presented again by MP Ciani, which will have to be discussed in Parliament on the points indicated, with an undertaking of responsibility by the Italia Government on the issue. In the meantime, and this really electrifies me, the interparliamentary group has worked on the **First Manifesto** of the rights and duties of the person with respiratory allergies. A real *Vademecum* that was presented on October 2 in the press room of the Chamber of Deputies.

The Manifesto has been translated into English, so that it can cross the borders of Italy, where this important initiative had its origin. You can find it attached in the Italian version at the end of the book. I am glad to share it with you so that you can be proud of it as I am.

The smile

"Butta Via i Fazzoletti" has not only helped stir the often-stagnant waters of politics, it has intrigued and entertained thousands of people with the "weird but true" stories of many allergic people and their way of finding a solution to the problem. These stories, which I have told in a humorous style, are absolutely true and are the fruit of the experience of Dr. Andrea di Rienzo Businco, an authoritative specialist in allergology and immunology, as well as a dear friend, who in addition to lending his pen to the preface of the book, contributed to its writing by telling the story of his life experiences in the doctor's surgery.

Stage adaptation

the sometimes grotesque stories with which people deal with the allergic pathology have also inspired the creation of a theatrical piece called *Humanit-as* by Lia Locatelli, producer, playwright and director of M.Art.E, Varese Performance Academy. Lia is an allergic patient and was immediately struck by the theme of the book. Her plays, moreover, are exquisitely social in nature. Who better than her could have transformed the book into a theatrical subject? This is how *Humanit-as was born*, a show in two acts that debuted as an absolute premiere in Varese on April 27, registering a sold-out despite the very long weekend scheduled in those days. Thus 200 people were thrown into a doctor's surgery, to listen to and live together with the protagonists the torment of the people of allergies, tissue always in hand, antihistamines and cortisone as life companions.

PREAMBLE

In this cross-section, everyone was able to see their habits depicted on stage, their behaviour that includes self-diagnosis and creative solutions adopted to deal with allergies. An original, engaging way to address a deep problem, often voiceless, that affects about 12 million people. Even the magazine "Più Salute e Benessere" issued by financial newspaper *Sole 24* dedicated two pages in the May issue to *Butta Via i Fazzoletti* and the message of dissemination that it carries forward. The book will be presented on October 18, in the Press Room of the Chamber of Deputies, in the presence of MP Paolo Ciani and Dr. Andrea di Rienzo Businco.

Not only that, but the book has also become international and speaks English with the title of NO MORE TISSUES. It goes beyond the Italian borders to find and create a European alliance on a theme that has been so overshadowed.

All this in just 700 days.

Again, THANK YOU, then, to all of you who have read my words, followed me on the Blog, who have been writing to me, who have taken part in the FB live broadcasts and have honoured me with their presence in the various meetings throughout Italy. Together we give voice to the people of allergies. THANK YOU to those who will read me and come to listen to me.

Who knows what will happen in the next 700 days.

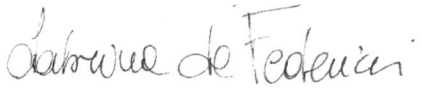

CHAPTER 1

A PLANET OF ALLERGIC PEOPLE

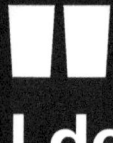

I decided to write this book specifically for them, for anyone who's tired of always walking around with tissues and drugs and is looking for a permanent solution.

CHAPTER 1 - A PLANET OF ALLERGIC PEOPLE

"Achoo!"

This is how for long, long years, my son said "good morning" to me every morning when I used to wake him up to go to school.

Not a "Hi mom", a "Ugh, 5 more minutes!" or a "I don't want to go today!". I've never enjoyed the typical dialogues that characterise the usual mother-child morning relationship during the school period.

I missed the pleasure of calling my son repeatedly to get him out of bed, while I often had to fight with the displeasure of hearing Simone start his day with a flurry of sneezes as soon as he woke up and seeing him jump up to sit up in bed while breathing heavily, emitting a terrifying whistle.

I had learned to keep a small Pantone sample book in my bag, just like an upholsterer or a painter would do, to identify which, among all the possible shades from red to purple, was the one my little one's skin and lips took on. Only in this way could I find my way around in the sea of medicines to use when, in between attacks of allergic rhinitis, atopic dermatitis and more or less violent asthma attacks, I had to decide in a matter of seconds whether to give him a common antihistamine, a cortisone-based medicine or to rush straight to the emergency room. Maybe this is why paint and varnish shops still give me shivers today.

With the arrival of Simone I entered, against my will, into the unknown world of allergies. Today my son's situation can no longer be defined problematic, but it still is – instead – for thousands of people, adults and children.

I decided to write this book specifically for them, for anyone who's tired of always walking around with tissues and drugs and is looking for a permanent solution.

The therapy that exists
(but that only few know about)

This has nothing to do with witchcraft, as some might think, given the lack of information on the subject, but rather about a curative therapy for allergies which pays the price of being, in fact, ignored.

This is the conclusion I came to following the statistics which show that the increase in allergic subjects – data provided by Istat [TN – Italian National Institute of Statistics] – does not correspond to an equal increase in the use of this therapy called *desensitization*.

There is no point in denying it: a patient who does not recover and continues to use antihistamines and cortisone-based drugs for their entire life is much more profitable for the market, which thus keeps "its customer" for life.

I'm just saying that, when I used to work as a medical rep, we were told what the motto of pharmaceutical companies is: "A long and sickly life".

Added to this is that allergists are often considered by the National

Health System to be less useful than other specialists. Proof of this is the fact that, when one of them retires, he is not replaced by a colleague: his hours are simply eliminated from the structure in which he worked or reconverted into other specialties.

This is why I decided to give wide visibility to the pathology, its course and its solution (which is already available on the market) through this book. A text that I strongly wanted to keep simple, clear and light, without making a scientific treatise manual out of it. Years ago, like many parents before and after me, I was groping in the dark, too, searching on the internet, like Diogenes with the lantern, for a miracle cure for my little one.

Since I landed in HAL Allergy, a pharmaceutical company that has been producing desensitization therapies since 1959, in order to allow the allergic patient to fight the annoying symptoms, as well as to get to the root of the problem.

People generally find out they have a type of allergic disease because they develop annoying symptoms – swelling, redness, sneezing, difficult breathing and many more – and they turn to an allergist to identify which substance is causing it.

At this point, drugs are usually prescribed – mostly antihistamines and cortisone-based in various forms – which act on the symptom by reducing its intensity, but certainly do not eliminate the cause. The problem lies right here.

It's fine to find an immediate remedy for the symptoms, but if it is not associated with a treatment that acts on the triggering causes, the allergic patient is destined to go from red to purple to bluish for the rest of their life.

The desensitization therapy is a process that lasts three years, at the end of which the clinical symptoms are significantly reduced. In fact, desensitization acts directly on the immune system, teaching it to recognize the external substance that causes the allergy.

The aim is to communicate to the body that the problem is not the triggering substance, but the anomaly in the immune system that pushes it to consider it "foreign" and, therefore, dangerous.

Rather than unleashing the usual war in which the enemy symptom is "fought", thanks to this therapy an alliance is created with the immune system to ensure that peace returns between it and the allergen.

Thus the subject can finally return to a natural lifestyle. In other words, the therapy becomes a "facilitator" of communication between a particularly wary immune system and Nature itself. Its purpose is precisely to create a dialogue and therefore an acceptance of mutual coexistence between the immune system and the wonderful environment in which it is immersed.

Allergens are substances that normally should not bother humans.

In some cases, however, a sudden sensitivity is triggered by one or more allergens in particular, developing various types of reactions.

Unfortunately this is not the worst aspect of allergies: there is the possibility that, if action is not taken in time, the subject goes from being monosensitive to polysensitive, i.e. suffering from more than one allergy – and they can also develop asthma, a disease from which there is no turning back: once you reach this stage you will have to live with it forever. It is the so-called "allergic march".

Thanks to the desensitization therapy, however, the symptoms disappear, allergies do not progress and there is no risk of developing allergic asthma.
"Am I still allergic?", Simone asked me after three years of therapy without sneezing.

Allergy is like a tattoo: the mark remains, but it lightens over time.
The body, which retains memory of the reactions developed towards substances perceived as enemies, confesses to being an allergic subject, but, in fact, the symptoms no longer exist. The early use of this therapy is very important for all allergy sufferers, but even more so for children, who have the precious opportunity to block the allergic progression.

If you are an allergic person or you also have children who suffer from this pathology, you will realize how incredibly important it is to prefer this therapy to classic drugs whose sole purpose is to temporarily silence the symptom (which – we know well – will return inevitably once the treatment is stopped).

The "everything and now"

Since, as I said before, there are few allergists in Italy, very few prescribe this treatment which is well known to them having been on the market for 30 years.

Why don't they propose it then?
The answer is not easy, there are several elements that combine with each other, exactly like in the process that triggers allergies.

Who is responsible for what?
In communication there is a specific law that explains that if the recipient does not understand the message, the fault lies with the sender.
Simple, you will tell me: then it's all the allergists' fault.

In most cases, the amount of work and the tight times of the visits lead the specialist to be quicker in their explanations and perhaps "less authoritative" towards the patients, who, for their part, want "everything right away" and want the symptoms to stop immediately.

I do understand this attitude because, as the mother of an allergic child – no longer a child but a boy – I used to take my beautiful Pantone of medicines out and about to intervene instantly. "Everything now" makes it more difficult for the allergist to communicate the duration of the desensitization therapy which, to be effective, requires at least three years. It is true that we are in the world of hit and run, but health is something precious that we must take care of ourselves first and foremost and give ourselves the time needed to achieve well-being results.

Above all we should realize that the relationship allergist/allergic patient represents a tandem that travels with the same rhythm and the victory of one represents the victory of the other. A tandem called therapeutic alliance which can proceed only if the patient continues the therapy for as long as necessary, without abandoning it before having achieved the goal, going on taking the necessary drugs when required and only if the specialist is ready to support and constantly check the goals achieved.

The statistics confirm both the difficulty of allergists in communicating the effectiveness and duration of the therapy on the one hand and that of patients – or parents of young patients – in understanding the extraordinary benefit that it brings: unfortunately 50% of the subjects involved decide to abandon the therapy during the first year, and this number reaches a peak of 70% in the second year.
The main reason is that the patient, on average, sees the first benefits after a few months and feels better, so he thinks it is not necessary to continue.

I understand the point, accustomed as they are to thinking according to the methods and times of the usual drugs but, by interrupting it early, not only do they fail to achieve the primary aim they had set themselves – desensitising the body towards an allergen – as it takes the immune system at least three years to achieve it, but this sudden decision also nullifies that initial improvement.

If you think about it, it is easy to understand how the immune system probably needs years to "convince" itself that the allergen in question is not an enemy, just as it took years to the body, and who knows how many, to develop that particular allergy.

The National Health System is also responsible

Another reason why this therapy is not as well-known as it should be, given the extraordinary results it guarantees, is that it is not supported by the National Health System.

The entire cost is borne by the patient, who cannot accept the idea of having to pay for a drug in a country where healthcare covers the majority of services and where antihistamines are available at negligible prices.

Unfortunately, this is a problem of our healthcare system which does not reimburse this therapy, despite being the only etiological therapy recognized by the World Health Organization (WHO); where etiological is not a "bad word" but indicates that the therapy treats the cause and not the symptom of allergies by reprogramming the immune system. Having been through it before you, I perfectly understand what you're thinking right now but I would like to make you evaluate one point: when you have to choose a new car, what do you take into consideration? Just the cost?

Or instead, do you think about what you will have to use it for, how long to keep it, reliability and safety, fuel consumption per km/l compared to a car that costs less?
In short, don't you weigh all the pros and cons before deciding which one to buy?
I'm sure you do, because we all do it every day, even when we go shopping at the supermarket and choose to buy some products because they are on offer, others because they are of good quality, others because they are organic or produced by the local farmer.

The same goes for the desensitization therapy: it makes sense to take on a cost once every three months for three years – as if you were leasing or buying an iPhone in instalments – to get rid of the symptoms that afflict you, once and for all, instead of spending much more and go on taking drugs all your life which, as we know, if they are good on one side can cause problems elsewhere due to side effects?
I'm sure you can answer that yourself!

Is it a vaccine?

Another aspect that I would like to clarify regarding this therapy arises from the questions that I constantly hear from those who approach me for information: is it a vaccine? Can I get this vaccine together with the first, second... millionth dose of the anti-Covid vaccine?

The desensitization therapy IS NOT A VACCINE against allergies. This is a misnomer because these are two vastly different things.

Let's consider the case of the Covid vaccine – given that it has been such a hot topic and it has been the biggest concern of those who have turned to me in recent months. The vaccine consists of a deactivated pathogen of the virus that is injected into a HEALTHY subject, so that the immune system is able to develop the antibodies necessary to fight the virus itself, in the event of contagion.

The desensitization therapy, on the other hand, is a real therapy, that is, it is used to treat a person ALREADY suffering from an allergy, to counteract a pathology ALREADY present in the body. It's a bit like saying that injecting heroin or a painkiller are the same thing just because, in both cases, you inject yourself.

The origins

The theory behind the desensitization therapy has very distant origins, just think of Mithridates, the ancient king of Pontus, who, being afraid of being poisoned, used to take small doses of snake venom to immunize himself. Now, even if today no one thinks they can be poisoned by the snakes that want to take away their throne – oh well, maybe someone does! – the principle is the same.

My aim is to inform people – including any Royals who feel at risk – about the importance of looking after their wellbeing when this is compromised by allergies.

Allergies are not to be underestimated

One of the key points why allergies are often scarcely considered or why there is little information on possible therapies to contrast them is linked to the perception that allergy is not a serious disease. This is because we connect the adjective *serious* to something lethal, while *serious* should also refer to the quality of life of a patient. If the latter has to give up going out, being among others, taking a walk in the park, playing five-a-side football or any other competitive sport, in short, the patient has to give up living, the quality of their life is so compromised that, yes, I think it is correct to speak of a serious pathology.

If we talk about children, the situation is even worse: paediatricians – the first to visit young patients – often invite parents not to intervene but to wait until the children grow up and the immune system is strengthened. Despite being in good faith, paediatricians are not experts in the field of allergies and, unintentionally, can cause damage, since by intervening late, that famous allergic march can be triggered and lead to more complex clinical situations as time passes.

Normally children are prescribed cortisone-based and antihistamine drugs via aerosol, to be taken constantly which not only do not solve the problem at its root, but trigger a series of consequences linked to the drugs themselves: cortisone acts on the kidneys and heart and both remedies cause an altered sense of hunger which inevitably leads to overweight and sometimes to less growth in height of the child himself.

There is prejudice, therefore, towards the desensitization therapy or the lack of knowledge of it or even the reticence to direct the child towards an allergy visit: the result is that children undergo therapies that stop the symptoms but not the allergy and, above all on the long period, they have side effects that can be important.

Furthermore, recognizing the child as an allergic subject, the paediatrician generally recommends prohibitions that lead this poor little creature to live under a glass dome: no dog, no cat, no park, no curtains or carpets; the mattress only if anti-mite, and so on. If the family already owns a pet, they advise them to get rid of it, adding a real mourning on the shoulders of a child who is growing up and should be free to behave like one.

This overprotection, which does not allow children to live in contact with nature, inevitably leads to overreactions when they accidentally come into contact with an animal or a plant.

Yes I know! As a mother I understand how difficult it is to make the right decision when it comes to your children. It is not easy to understand what is best to do and who to listen to.

It is precisely for this reason, having been there before you, that, with this book, I want to give you all the information you need to make your decision, with the peace of mind of having examined all the hypotheses.

Another aspect that is little considered when talking about allergies is that the mucous membranes of the nose become hypertrophic in allergic subjects.

This is a serious problem because the mucosa that internally lines the nose is the same as that found in the rest of the body – for example at the tracheal, pharyngeal and lung levels – and, ultimately, it too is damaged. If the mucosa is damaged, the effectiveness of the human body's first defensive barrier is reduced.

I emphasize all this to counter the tendency to consider allergies as a minor problem, even on the part of allergy sufferers themselves who sometimes prefer to "plug the hole" with a hit-and-run therapy – the antihistamine – which does not provide a solution to the underlying problem, instead of engaging in a definitive treatment that brings many benefits to the quality of life. If it is true that the number of deaths due to cardiological or oncological pathologies cannot be compared to that due to allergies, it is also true that every year deaths are also recorded due to anaphylactic shocks or very violent asthmatic attacks caused by allergens such as lichwort.

Therefore, why not choosing a desensitization therapy that treats the triggers of the allergy instead of a symptom suppressor that will never lead to the solution?

I am convinced that to live well we must take care of ourselves and our body in the best possible way and this therapy allows us to prevent future serious problems caused by allergies and asthma.

The time factor

Of course, the desensitization therapy requires discipline and commitment – since it lasts three years – because it consists of administering to the patient the allergen that causes the allergic reaction in minimal doses.

The administration must be carried out slowly, in very small doses, to avoid the violent reactions mentioned above.

In fact, in cases of pollen allergy – since this therapy applies to any type of inhalant – the dosages are often reduced during the pollen season, taking into account the sum of the pollen that is administered with that with which the patient makes contact with in nature.
In the case, for example, of an allergy to cats, different therapies are applied depending on whether there is a cat in the house or not: if there is not, the therapy can be carried out in the established doses, but if the animal lives in the house it is necessary to administer smaller doses of allergens to avoid the cumulative action of the two,

with a possible consequent anaphylactic shock. In the latter case the dosage is very low and the patient is constantly monitored.

The truth is that with the desensitization therapy it is possible to cure any type of allergy due to inhalants or bee/wasp stings because this is modelled on the patient based on their needs and the lifestyle they lead. In this regard – remaining on the animal topic – I remember a beautiful girl, whom we helped with this desensitisation therapy, who practically spent her life hugging her German shepherd and had developed an allergy to the dog fur: with discipline and patience you can do everything.

The message I would like to convey clearly with this book is that, unlike what is normally thought, allergies can be cured and it is not necessary to live with them all your life, seeing your conditions or those of your children worsen as time goes by.

Allergy is a chronic and disabling pathology but we can choose to follow a therapy that I could define as "semi-chronic" since it lasts three years and not a lifetime and treats the triggering causes, not the acute phase.

There is a big difference between following a therapy for only three years and suffering from allergies for your whole life. It is true that the concept of time is different for each of us, but three years compared to an average lifespan of 80 represents 4% of all the years available to us.

The feedback obtained by committing for this time is enormously more advantageous than all the strategies used and the effort made to solve the problem.

Who I am

Before leaving you undisturbed to read this book, here is some information about me, just to let you know in what circumstance I decided to write it.

The professional path that led me to become Country Manager of HAL Allergy starts from afar. I was born in the Marche region, I belong to Abruzzo and I am Roman by adoption, and grew up with the desire, since I was at the high school, to attend the School of Journalism in Milan and become a scientific populariser.

Milan seemed very far away and my parents' reaction to my possible move to Milan was so disproportionate, at times exaggerated if not even ridiculous, that I ended up attending the faculty of Natural Sciences in Rome and graduating in Palaeontology.

A palaeontologist on loan to the pharmaceutical industry

If you are wondering why palaeontology, the answer is that I have always been interested in the human race, in its biological evolution and it seemed to me to be the right faculty to understand the present through the reasons of the past and the development of man. What does palaeontology have to do with allergies? I could answer that it played the role of the classic sliding doors.

The PhD I was granted was not enough to support myself financially and I didn't want to go back home to my parents: so I looked for a job.

I applied for a position as a medical-scientific reps without knowing, in practice, anything about the job, only following my mantra that everything can be learned and that in life it is not a question of "if" but only of "when".

I didn't know what a medical representative exactly did but I am extroverted, enthusiastic and with a natural propensity to interact with people and establish a relationship with them.

I'm also curious and this has always helped me a lot. They were truly instructive and above all fun years: I changed various companies, I was faced with different roles until I landed in a brand-new company, one that is normally defined a "startup" and which today is a very important multinational company, known to everyone for its first drug approved against Covid, Gilead.

At Gilead I developed my entire career, from hospital informant to area manager and, finally, Italian sales director. That company was a jewel. I left it in 2008 following the retirement of my general manager, nephew of the writer Gianni Rodari and an enlightened person belonging to Modena's intellectual class, who was able to create an incredible pharmaceutical reality, thanks above all to the trust he placed in his managers.

I worked very well with him and always had *carte blanche* in my decisions, which allowed me to interpret the role of sales director, generally "rigid", in a creative way, and more in line with my eclectic nature.

A role which, however, involves interaction with people, with doctors, with many different interlocutors and where the ability to know how to communicate plays a fundamental role.

And this is why in 2009 I enrolled in a three-year master course in media-communication counselling: *trait d'union* between the passion for homo sapiens and journalism.

After a brief three-year stint in a pharmaceutical market research company (I just couldn't stay away from that sector) I returned to the other side of the fence with the company I still work for today, HAL Allergy, a biotechnology company specializing in desensitization therapies against allergies.

Old loves, however, are never forgotten and the passion for writing has led me to collaborate with various online publications and blogs; for a long period I wrote for the columns "La finestra – storie di belle realtà" [TN – The window – stories of beautiful realities] and "La sublime etica del gusto" [TN – The sublime ethics of taste] for which I still write occasionally.

From here I started to give a precise imprinting to my future work, based on active listening and empathy, because for me "human resonance" is an essential value. Even within my role, "sales" is not the final goal: the most important thing is to establish a relationship with customers, get in tune with them and thus be able to offer them what they really need.

Still not satisfied and being interested in nutrition since the time of my thesis in Paleontology, specific on the paleo-nutrition of an ancient population of Geli – a site in central Sudan – I enrolled in a master course in Gastronomic Counselling and, later, in one in Food and Wine Journalism, always pursuing that initial "dream".

Each experience enriches my personal and I would say professional background, where I constantly experiment with what I learn.

At this point in my journey, all that was missing was the book I had reflected upon so many times, a book that would help all those who suffer from allergies to improve their lives.

"No more tissues" perfectly expresses my aspiration: to offer an opportunity of choice – and therefore of liberation – to all those who do not yet know that there is a desensitization therapy that solves the problem of allergies by treating the cause.

The book tells about real cases – however particular – and the healing path that led them all to live better "without tissues".
Enjoy the reading!

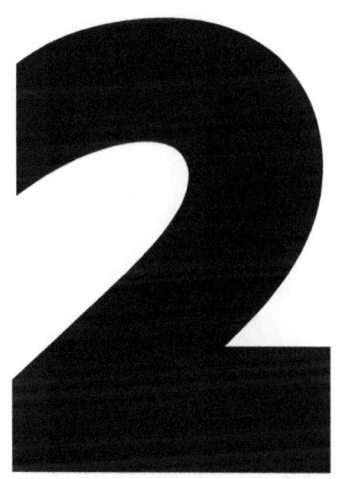

CHAPTER 2 – Case History

THE PLANE, THE PILOT AND THE CAT

> During the flight
> my nose had swollen,
> and the itching had
> become stronger
> and stronger,
> it had also spread
> to my throat and,
> in addition to sneezing,
> I was coughing
> violently.

CHAPTER 2 – CASE HISTORY: THE PLANE, THE PILOT AND THE CAT

The morning had started splendidly: the horoscope predicted a fantastic week and, considering that I would have to fly a Boeing 737 from Rome to Dublin and then enjoy a nice evening at Temple Bar with some friends, I had no doubts about it.

In short, I couldn't wait to lock myself in the cockpit and fly pleasantly to my destination. That day Lorenzo was my co-pilot and when I got on board, I found him already sitting in his seat while carrying out the necessary checks.

– Have you started the engine? – I joked.

– Absolutely. A gorgeous redhead is waiting for me tonight in Dublin! What are your plans? – he exclaimed.

– I'll go have a beer!

– Fantastic. Let's fire up this beast, Maverick!

The flight attendants were boarding the travellers, we were almost there: "Dublin, I'm coming" I said to myself, "Tonight, I'm not going to miss a pint of Guinness for anything in the world, poured as they can only do in Ireland."

Once the boarding was completed, I made my announcement to the passengers and closed the loudspeaker, ready to take off. I had just given full power to the engines when a ferocious itch in my nose made me sneeze.

Once. Twice. Three times.

Lorenzo turned to look at me:

– Is everything okay, Giorgio?

– Yes fine. Well, there must be something in the air – I said, dusting off the old-fashioned idea that my grandmother used to maintain with great confidence, especially when someone sneezed several times in a row.

Even if, in the end, that "something" that was in the air represented for everyone a mysterious element, something mythological, with an impenetrable nature. During the flight my nose had swollen, and the itching had become stronger and stronger, it had also extended to my throat and in addition to sneezing, I was coughing violently.

Lorenzo ventured a hypothesis: – It must be the dust. After all, we breathe regenerated air. After a two-and-a-half-hour flight (it takes three hours and forty minutes to get to Dublin) I was completely transformed: I was looking more and more like Godzilla, and it was certainly not a pleasant sight to look at. I couldn't wait to get off for some fresh air.

That was the first time my allergy kicked in. Later, during some rather short flights, the symptoms had presented themselves very mildly, so much so that I had taken into consideration the possibility to contact an allergist who could verify my sensitivity to a specific allergen. I had reviewed my entire clinical life and couldn't remember to have had allergies in 35 years! But why right now?

The family doctor, when I told him what had happened, expressed himself peremptorily:

– Giorgio, you should contact an allergist to check for any sensitivity...

– But no, doctor! – I replied boldly – there were few sneezes, I had a more severe episode only once, but it never happened again. It probably was a coincidence.

I also borrowed the philosophy of "it must have been a coincidence" from my grandmother – I didn't feel like condemning her, poor thing: she lived in the mountains, there were no pharmacies and most ailments were cured with ancient home practices – however, my grandmother's inference "it must have been a coincidence" had collapsed miserably during a flight from Rome to New York: 9 hours and 55 minutes.

After going to the bathroom to rinse my face – I don't want to dwell on the anxious expression of the passengers when they saw me coming out of the cabin while sneezing, with red spots on my neck and shortness of breath – I was back to my seat. After a few minutes, the symptoms returned, stronger than before: tears, coughing, sneezing for over an hour straight, in the end I almost fainted on the control board.

Once back in Rome, after a nightmare return flight, I had definitively filed my grandmother's philosophy and reluctantly made an appointment with Doctor Di Rienzo Businco.

The study was sober, furnished with antique furniture that made the wait pleasant. The environment did not absolutely give the impression of a place attended by sick people, but rather showed a certain flair. I don't know why at a certain point I sighed with relief and calmed down.

This must be someone who knows his job, I told myself, and after formulating that elementary thought, I immediately felt better. I was already thinking that maybe that visit wasn't that necessary after all, since I hadn't had any symptoms for a few days, when Doctor Businco called me in.

– Confess: you wanted to leave, sir…

He began smiling, with that relaxed attitude, like someone who knows what he's doing and listens to you carefully. And not just with his ears.

– Giorgio. My name is Giorgio and… well… Yes, I thought about it, actually – I replied a little embarrassed.

He smiled again, amused.

– So, on the phone you told me that you are a sportsman, you don't smoke, have a regular diet, have never had any allergy problems but these days you are experiencing very strong symptoms at work. Is that correct?

– Exactly, doctor. I really don't understand: I'm a pilot, I'm locked in the cabin all the time and the air is pressurized… – Yes, on the surface it might seem safe to you, but allergies are insidious pathologies that can appear suddenly, and at any age. In the meantime, let's carry out some prick tests and then, if necessary, we will investigate further.

He uncovered my arm and applied a series of allergens to my skin: a long line that reminded me of a landing strip. 15 minutes of waiting and a nice red bump came out, of a truly surprising size.

– Good news, we found the culprit! Do you have a cat? – asked the doctor.

– Absolutely not, I don't have time for pets, if you consider my job…

– I replied rolling my eyes.

– Excellent, you are actually allergic to cat fur! – He reiterated with determination.

– But I just told you that I don't have a cat… – I replied discouraged.

– Yes, you told me, but it's not your "non-cat". What triggers your allergy are those owned by the thousands of passengers that are welcomed on your plane, on every flight.

In front of my perplexed expression or, rather, my widened eyes, the doctor went on:

– The cat allergen is particularly insidious, the animal's fur remains on clothes, sofas, objects, even for years. You would be amazed to know how many invisible cats got on your plane; this is why you show symptoms on a plane, even if there are no cats on board, because you are in contact with that allergen for many hours.

The longest flights are the most disastrous for you, aren't they?

I felt anguish grip my throat and in a strangled voice I croaked:

– Are you telling me that I have to stop flying?

He smiled as he began to write something in the prescription pad.

– Of course not! You just need to take care of yourself appropriately and have patience; it's a long therapy that requires discipline and continuity, but you must have plenty of discipline considering your job – he consoled me as he handed me out the sheet with the prescription.

So I started carrying my vial of sublingual desensitization therapy with me in every flight, initiating a ritual: check of the equipment, engine start and five drops under the tongue. Take off!

During one of the usual trips to Prague, Carlo, one of my co-pilots, as we crossed Wenceslas Square to reach the hotel, took me by the arm and asked me:

– Giorgio, have you solved your allergy issue? I would like to talk to you about it.

– I am being treated by a very good doctor, I am recovering through a specific treatment, it takes some time but I am feeling already better.

– I don't doubt it, but come and visit my wife's allergist too. He is number one. She solved all her problems and this changed her life, trust me.

– Thank you, you are kind, but I have full faith in mine!

– I understand, but he's not like my wife's, trust me. He is the best in the field – insisted Carlo.

– Look, I wouldn't change Doctor Di Rienzo Businco for nothing in the world – I replied almost annoyed.

– Doctor Businco? – he asked me – Andrea Di Rienzo Businco?

– Sure! He is my allergist.

– I wanted to recommend him to you! – Carlo said laughing – My wife started living a normal life again after following his treatment!

We burst out laughing at the incredible coincidence as we approached the reception desk.

Today I can as well say that my life has changed, in many ways. I go on flying without the problems I had before and at home, waiting for my return, there is a wonderful, very hairy, red cat.

I found him wandering around my house for a week, looking for food.

He lives with me now, his name is Iceman.

Maverick, of course, is me.

PRECIOUS PILL N.1

Allergies can occur even without direct exposure to the allergen.

It is advisable, in the presence of typical symptoms, to always carry out some tests to exclude and confirm the allergic pathology and, in case of a positive response, to immediately start an adequate desensitization therapy.

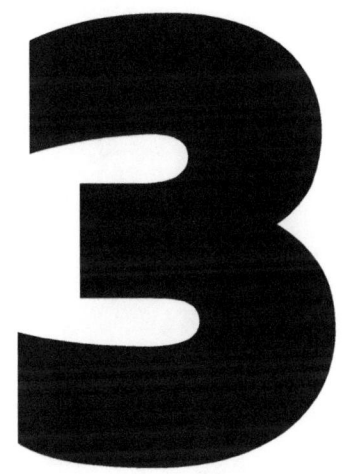

CHAPTER 3 – Case History

THE LAWYER AND THE LICHWORT

> This had been my life until a few months earlier when, with the sudden blossoming of spring, I began to feel a terrible itch in my nose during my walks.

CHAPTER 3 – CASE HISTORY: THE LAWYER AND THE LICHWORT

After over 40 years of practicing law, I was enjoying retirement. My day was scheduled by a precise and very pleasant routine. Early in the morning I used to take Barolo, my wonderful dachshund and lifelong companion, out for a walk, together with his son, a 9-month-old puppy I had named Prezzemolo [Parsley]. Don't ask me the origin of this weird name, because it was my wife's idea. Perhaps she borrowed it from her passion for cooking, given the little one's ability to be anywhere, exactly like this herb.

After leaving the profession of lawyer and after my children had embarked on their own path, I was still living with Anna in our small apartment in Via Veneto: from there, three times a day, I delighted in a walk around Porta Pinciana together with my two dachshunds.

At seven in the morning, after waving goodbye to the porter – and having slalomed between the floor rag and her super-polishing and ultra-slippery wax for which I had a real terror – I loved walking at a slow pace towards the stone walls that surround the city.

This had been my life until a few months earlier when, with the sudden blossoming of spring, during my walks, I began to feel a terrible itch in my nose followed by inexplicable bursts of sneezing which also caused me some embarrassment.

The first time it had happened I hadn't given it much thought, thinking it was a coincidence, even though the itching had reappeared during the afternoon walk and also in the evening. On the second day, the episode occurred again and more intensely, so much so that, when

I met my neighbour, we took the opportunity to have a coffee at the bar in an attempt to stop the sneezing and the annoying cough that was tormenting me for a few minutes.

I remember that that evening I talked about it with my wife Anna.

– What could it be, you might have a bit of a cold, Luciano! – she told me lightly, shrugging her shoulders.

– A cold doesn't go away if I go indoors or into a bar, does it? After all, it's spring, what if I were allergic to something?

– At your age? Forget about it! – And she ended the conversation like that.

Life went on peacefully but Barolo, Prezzemolo and I had started exchanging curious points of view during our walks, because, strangely, Barolo had also started to sneeze every time we passed by the Aurelian walls.

Prezzemolo looked at us astonished and none of us three could explain what was happening.

– In your place, I would make an appointment at the doctor's. Maybe you're about to die – Barolo told me one day, waging his tail from side to side with a thoughtful expression.

– For a few sneezes and some itchy eyes? – I echoed him, perplexed.

CHAPTER 3 – CASE HISTORY: THE LAWYER AND THE LICHWORT

– Why not? – sighed Prezzemolo with wide puppy eyes – if you die it will a catastrophe, who do you leave us with, with Anna? She doesn't buy biscuits filled with beef pâté, I don't want to be alone with Anna.

– Boy, it seems premature to bury me because of two sneezes and a bit of itching, don't you think? – I said.

– You never know – Barolo replied – make an appointment. And let's see what Dr. Giacomello has to say.

– The vet?

– Oh, sure. What if the allergy was contagious? Haven't you seen how many times I sneeze, too? Do you want to see me dead? – Barolo was looking a bit melodramatic. I don't know why he reminded me of those 1950s films with Rock Hudson. The black and white ones.

– May I know what happened to you today? You two look like jinxes!

Anyway, yes, you sneeze too, Barolo. How strange… – I replied doubtfully.

– Oh, I told you. I'm going to die," he replied, shaking his head.

– Why don't you take him to an analyst instead of the vet? – proposed Prezzemolo.

Our walk ended with handkerchiefs and red eyes, punctuated by a dry cough. A few days later, during dinner Anna looked at me worriedly: I had a red nose, swollen eyes and a whooping dry cough.

– You can't go on like this. We should talk to the family doctor and see what he advises us to do.

– Otherwise he is going to die! – Barolo barked from the armchair, in a panic.

– I'm not dying! – I shouted, turning towards my hysterical-depressed dachshund.

– Are you angry with the dog, Luciano? Who are you talking to?

– Of course not, I'm not talking to anyone, dear – I swiftly defended myself, looking at Barolo in a trance.

The next day our doctor was clear: I had to consult an allergist because the symptoms that afflicted me seemed due to an allergy and it was appropriate to undergo some tests.

– See? Maybe we will survive and not all die. – Barolo rejoiced when Anna, on the advice of a friend, had made an appointment at the office of Doctor Di Rienzo Businco.... –

– Why two doctors? Then it's serious... – said Barolo – I would go to either Doctor Di Rienzo or Doctor Businco, you have to rely on just one doctor! And also, call the vet, because I sneeze and feel an itchy nose too, just like you – my dog went on, sitting next to me on the sofa.

– Can you stop with this attitude? You'll see – I'll find a solution. Doctor Di Rienzo Businco, who has two names but is only one person, is very good. Anna was told that he is the best in the field.

– Yes, but as a precaution I would like you to buy the beef-filled biscuits first. So, just to be sure, it's not that I don't trust doctors, eh ... – Prezzemolo intervened from its basket in front of us.

– You're putting on a few kilos, son – hissed Barolo – if you don't stop, the next ones will be diet biscuits.

Two days later I paid a visit to Doctor Di Rienzo Businco and underwent tests. Result: allergic to lichwort, a very insidious weed that grows on the stone walls in tufts and which in some subjects causes the onset of allergies with rather severe symptoms.

My case was certainly not among the most serious, but I urgently needed a pharmacological therapy that would soothe the symptoms and give me back the pleasure of my daily walks.

I was truly amazed by the fact that up until the age of 73 I had never suffered from even a slight intolerance and suddenly, from one day to the next, I discovered I was allergic.

Doctor Di Rienzo Businco proposed me a desensitization therapy, explaining that I would have to be strict in taking it every day and very patient, precisely in the sense of having a lot of patience.

In fact, the symptoms then began to ease month after month until, after about three years, they disappeared completely. Now I have started enjoying my retired life and trips out of town with my wife and my two talkative quadrupeds.

The walks with Barolo and Prezzemolo have once again become a moment of relaxation and we trot at full speed along the Aurelian walls up to Villa Borghese, without the shadow of a sneeze.

Ah! I took Barolo to the vet: he wasn't allergic, he was just stressed. Once I recovered, he stopped sneezing, too.

I put Prezzemolo on a diet instead, but that's another story.

PRECIOUS PILL N.2

Allergies can appear suddenly, without being preceded by "useful signals", and at any age.

There is no precise age in which to develop reactions to allergens of any type.

In the presence of symptoms, the assumption "I have never suffered from it before" is not an "insurance" on health.

At any age, whenever the classic symptoms of an allergic reaction appear, it is advisable to contact an allergist for further information.

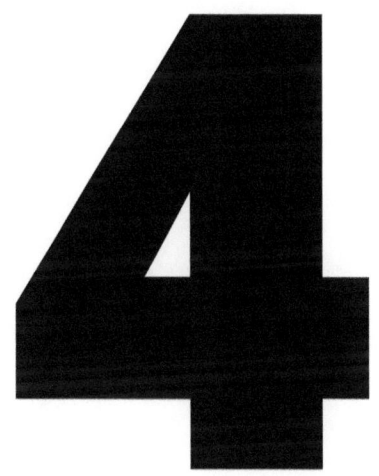

CHAPTER 4 – Case History

HIM, HER AND THE CATS

> "I couldn't be happier. However, I didn't know yet that problems were waiting for me just around the corner.

CHAPTER 4 – CASE HISTORY: HIM, HER AND THE CATS

It didn't seem real to me: I had won her over. She, Silvia, was the most beautiful woman in the world to me. For over six months, and with a certain dedication – and a fair margin of desperation as well – I had pursued her with assiduity and romanticism. That period had been a waltz of red roses delivered to her home, tickets for the trendiest plays, charming little surprises, like a 160 euro bottle of wine (you know what I mean) brought for a "casual" spaghetti dinner at some of her friends' place.

The moment in which I declared my feelings to her was the most beautiful of my life: Silvia, smiling, threw her arms around my neck and gave me a kiss. As soon as I got home, I told everything to Mario and Milo, my two cats, my best friends. We have lived together for over six years and I had never left them for a moment: we were living in symbiosis and sometimes I spoke about them as if they were people.

With an aura of unapproachable Egyptian deities they listened to me sprawled on the sofa. Milo, the more impatient of the two, grumbled and looked away while I was delirious in my description of my beloved:

– Guys, you have no idea! Silvia is wonderful, stunning, elegant. I couldn't imagine another woman by my side! She's a bit, how to say... well, like Duchess of the Aristocats, you know?

My two big cats showed me their behinds and nonchalantly approached the bowl of kibbles.

NO MORE TISSUES SABRINA DE FEDERICIS

My partner and I had started seeing each other regularly and our love story was taking the shape of a life project. I couldn't be happier than this. However, I didn't know yet that the problems were waiting for me just around the corner.

The day Silvia was supposed to move into my apartment in the centre of Rome, I couldn't wait to cook for her and prepare a perfect dinner. I had also set a magnificent table on our terrace, overlooking the Colosseum. The sunset illuminated the entire living room, and the aperitif was ready when she entered the house with her suitcases.

As soon as she got into the living room, she performed a high note that not even Maria Callas in her best days could have played.

I turned around and jolted.

– Silvia? What's happening? Is everything okay?

– Cats! Giulio, you have cats! – she exclaimed, upset.

– Yes, I told you…

– No! You told me that you had two friends from whom you have never split off: Mario and Milo. My God… are they cats?

– Sure! My cats. They are adorable, very calm, they won't bother you at all, you'll see! They don't even scratch! – Giulio, this is not the problem. I am allergic to cats, their hair, I don't know what else... since I was a child: believe me, I am at risk of having serious problems if I stay here.

I tried to play down, to tell her that over time, perhaps, her allergy had lost the intensity it had when she was a child.

– Let's try and see how it goes, darling. Don't cross your bridges before you come to them.

After about five minutes I realized that something was happening and certainly not what I had in mind. Silvia began to feel unwell, to have a itch in her throat, nose and eyes, which were watering abundantly.

My woman – it was clear – in those conditions she wouldn't have been able to move in with me and my cats. It looked like a nightmare.

Unfortunately Silvia had not underestimated the matter at all. After about half an hour, in fact, she began to sneeze, then at night, despite leaving the cats in the adjoining room, her breathing became laboured and her allergic rhinitis gave her no rest.

At that point there was no other solution than to make a call to my friend Andrea Di Rienzo Businco, a highly trained allergist whose skills, by pure luck, I had never benefited from until that day. I remember calling him in a panic in order to make an appointment for Silvia, because the situation had turned quite serious.

Andrea was very clear: my partner would have had to undergo a personalized desensitization therapy based on the allergen that caused the reaction, which would have led to the complete solution of the problem, but during the period of treatment I would have had to choose: either Silvia or the cats. As a matter of fact, the presence of cats during the desensitization therapy would have boosted the strength of the allergen.

I didn't know what to do. I loved Silvia but Mario and Milo were my family, a part of me and my life, an appendix without which I would have never been the same. I looked at them heartbroken while they swayed their tails slowly, almost as if to exert a hypnotic effect. It was precisely at that moment that I found the solution: renting a second apartment!

My wonderful cats would have had a house of their own where they could reign over everything while I would have moved with Silvia, for the entire period of the treatment, to another apartment.

I shuttled between our apartment and the "Cats' Manor" for three years, during which Silvia regularly followed the desensitization therapy in drops and showed a constant improvement.

In the end, after her complete recovery, we finally returned, happily, to my apartment with a view on the Colosseum. My cats, needless to say, were exactly where I had left them.

PRECIOUS PILL N.3

Allergies, if neglected, can trigger a "cascade" mechanism called "allergic march", involving multiple organs and districts of the body to the point of prompting intense reactions such as breathing crises.

Consulting an allergist and starting a desensitization therapy, without limiting yourself to suppressing the symptom, is the right approach to the allergic pathology, in order to take the path to recovery.

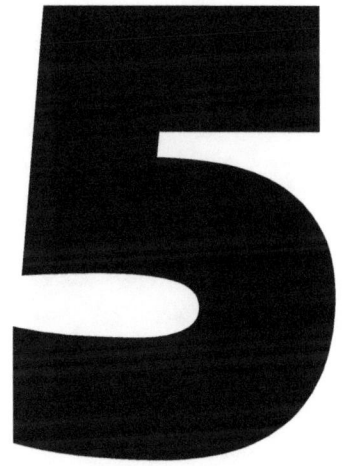

CHAPTER 5 – Case History

OBSTACLE JUMPING

> She was breathing, no doubt, but something was wrong. She felt like she was taking in less air than usual and that her muscles were not ready to sprint despite the warm-up.

CHAPTER 5 – CASE HISTORY: OBSTACLE JUMPING

Miriam was ready: she was loosening her muscles up and breathing rhythmically to prepare for the race while waiting for the signal to start the competition.

She was breathing, no doubt, but something was wrong. She felt like she was taking in less air than usual and that her muscles were not ready to sprint despite the warm-up.

She caressed Raphael, the magnificent horse and companion on adventures, and she bent over him to speak in his ear:

– Let's show them who we are!

She smiled at the movement of her steed's muzzle as it seemed to nod at her words. She raised her face to the sky, closed her eyes and let herself be flooded by the May sun, trying to capture the energy needed for the upcoming race.

She had prepared well, she had trained more than usual, yet she felt a bit of restlessness within herself.

Maybe it's time to stop – thought Miriam reluctantly – after all I'm 40 years old. What do I expect?

Much more, she answered herself sincerely.

After all, she was competing in her age category and the other contestants were her age, so what was wrong?

The judge gave the signal and she left those thoughts behind.

She took a deep breath, focused on the obstacles in front of her and told herself "One at a time, as always."

She nodded elegantly and walked to the start of the obstacle course that awaited her. She spurred her horse and set off, showing her typical grace.

She jumped the obstacles, one after another, concentrating only on the course.

After each leap she focused on the next one with her senses alert to detect every slight change in the animal beneath her.

She finished the race route tired and not completely satisfied: it had taken too long.

She turned to look at the scoreboard: she was seventh, but three competitors still had to take to the track.

She leaned forward, stroked the horse gently and whispered to him:

– Raphael, my friend, this time I made you lose. I'm getting old…

– What are you saying? You're in great shape, haven't you seen how the stableboy buzzes around you when you take me to the pits? –

The white-footed horse seemed to respond by shaking its muzzle and making a noise that actually reminded a raspberry.

– What now, are you kidding me? Who ever looked at him! And anyway, we lost because of me...

– Maybe it's because you've put on a few extra pounds, in fact my back hurts a bit, I'll get scoliosis...

Miriam started laughing despite the situation, but that sense of general unease was still there. She inhaled air and disappointment and headed towards the pits, where Federico, her coach, was waiting for her.

As she walked away from the race, her frustration grew: When did it start? When did her performances start to get worse?

In December she had finished first, setting a new time record.

How was it possible that just four months later she couldn't even place in the top three?

– Don't worry – said Federico – everyone has a bad day.

– Is it just this?

– Don't even think about it. You've never been so fit.

– The result says otherwise.

– You've been doing this sport too long to let a single negative result affect you.

– Yes, but something is wrong.

– And we will understand what it is.

Miriam took her tissue out of her pocket and blew her nose. – You didn't seem to have a cold this morning – said the coach, noticing Miriam's red eyes.

– No, that's true, but my nose itches. There is something that bothers me.

– You might be allergic to something – Federico theorized.

A glimmer of hope crossed Miriam's eyes.

– Could this explain the drop in the performance?

The coach thought about it for a moment.

– If I remember correctly, last year something similar happened in spring.

CHAPTER 5 – CASE HISTORY: OBSTACLE JUMPING

– You're not helping me – sighed Miriam – reminding me of my failures won't cheer me up for the next race.

– Maybe. What if you're allergic to pollen or something else that comes out in spring? If you think about it, last year was also the only occasion in which you didn't perform at your best...

A hopeful smile appeared on Miriam's face.

– It's worth investigating!

Miriam went to see the allergist even though she had never suffered from allergies in the past.

– Doctor, maybe it's nothing – she tried to play down – maybe it's just age and I have to accept the fact that it's time to retire; nevertheless I wanted to give it a try before giving up the sport I love. I'm sorry because I train a lot, maybe even more than before, but my racing times are getting longer.

– I can't tell you now whether the drop in performance is linked to some type of allergy or not – replied Doctor Di Rienzo Businco – but from the symptoms you describe to me I would hypothesize so, I would certainly focus more on an allergen than on age. The tests will give us the answer.

Doctor Di Rienzo Businco carried on the prick tests on her and Miriam turned out to be allergic to grasses. The allergy was induced by the inhalation of pollen grains dispersed in the environment, also present on the competition fields where Miriam raced.

The symptoms, in fact, appeared recurrently in the months of the year in which the plant flowered, generally between March and September. Miriam began a desensitization therapy – which is still ongoing – and even in the last season she achieved excellent results in the spring competition: after the race, even before dismounting from the horse, she called Doctor Di Rienzo Businco, enthusiastic:

– Doctor! I came second! Not a matter of old age! – And she burst out laughing.

Meanwhile, Raphael was showing off an elegant dressage gait as it headed towards her shelter, as if wanting to strut his stuff.

Miriam caressed its neck and out of the corner of her eye she saw the stableboy waiting for her with the stall door open: he was a handsome boy, tall and strong.

She straightened her back, fixed her hair and took a – finally deep – breath.

Why not, she said to herself, after all I'm still a girl...

PRECIOUS PILL N.4

When the allergic pathology shows up through breathing difficulties, it interferes with performance in competitive and non-competitive sporting activities.

In collaboration with CONI, protocols are being developed for Olympic athletes, which will soon be tested on the field with the Paddle team.

By improving nasal breathing even slightly, it was found that athletes are able to lower their times by even a second, an enormity at high levels, where hundredths of a second make the difference between getting on the podium or staying behind.

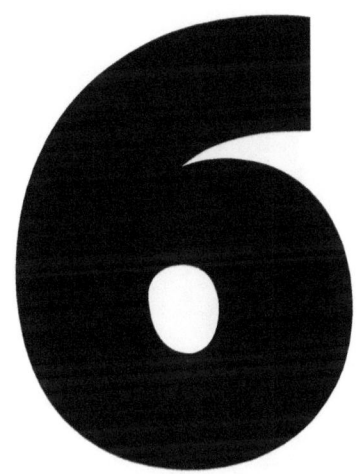

CHAPTER 6 – Case History

THE UNDERWATER LAWYER

> He looked at himself in the mirror again and sighed: once again he had to go to the office to meet his customers, trying to hide the problem that made him so uncomfortable.

CHAPTER 6 – CASE HISTORY: THE UNDERWATER LAWYER

The alarm clock began to crackle. Giulio reached out a hand and after two, three attempts he managed to turn it off. He wouldn't be able to avoid four court hearings that morning. He stretched for a long time, gave a good yawn and, after getting up, went to the bathroom.

He took off his pyjamas, adjusted the chromotherapy shower head and the temperature, took the mask and snorkel from the bathroom cabinet and put them on. He looked at himself in the mirror: naked wearing a diving mask – it wasn't a great sight. I can't go on like this, he said to his reflection, shaking his head. The tube, or rather the snorkel, swayed with him. By now he had become an expert in diving equipment like a diver of the Fire Brigade.

He got into the shower, taking care not to wet the aerator and not be forced to take off his mask due to coughing, thus allowing the water to hurt his face.

Water.

Being allergic to water sucks! – he exclaimed as he used the knob to adjust the intensity of the blue jet coming down from the shower head.

Once the shower was over he freed his face from that torture and dried himself.

Even though he was always very careful, his dermatitis showed no signs of decrease: he was red on his temples and forehead, at the hairline, and the small whitish skins that raised when he rubbed himself with the towel reminded him of Pop's scales, his wife's goldfish, who had died of old age the week before.

His head itched as if he hadn't washed in a month even though he had just finished shampooing. With two fingers he took a little nourishing cream and applied it to the affected area. He was massaging his forehead lightly when his wife entered the bathroom:

– Are you done? Can I take a shower?

– Of course – he replied, embarrassed at having been caught red-handed.

In fact, his wife, after realizing that she was using her cream, addressed him:

– Again? Why don't you buy your own instead of finishing mine!

Then she let the bathrobe slide onto the carpet and entered the shower stall.

In another moment he would have reacted to his wife's provocation but in that moment, he couldn't think of anything other than that damn dermatitis!

He looked at himself in the mirror again and sighed: once again

CHAPTER 6 – CASE HISTORY: THE UNDERWATER LAWYER

he had to go to the office to meet his customers, trying to hide the problem that made him so uncomfortable.

He decided to look up on the internet once again, hoping to find a remedy for his allergy. Then he brightened up and instead started looking for an allergist to make an appointment with. The next day he went to Doctor Di Rienzo Businco's office – he had been very kind and had agreed to receive him as the latest patient given the urgency – with the hope of being able to find a solution. After a few minutes of waiting, he was invited to sit down.

– Doctor, I have this dermatitis that never goes away. It bothers me a lot and it's not nice to look at. When I'm at work, I notice customers staring at me and I feel uncomfortable – said he, all in one breath.

– I understand – nodded the doctor – first let's try to understand what it is and then...

He couldn't finish the sentence before Giulio interrupted him.

– Doctor, I already know what I'm allergic to! I'm allergic to water!

Doctor Di Rienzo Businco remained unperturbed.

– How did you identify the cause? – He asked in a neutral voice.

– It's simple – replied Giulio – because I get it when I touch water. Especially when I take a shower.

– Have you ever had allergy tests? – insisted the doctor.

– No, but I found a temporary solution even if it doesn't work very well and is also very annoying...

– What is it about?

– Well, Doctor, it may seem strange to you, but I shower with my diving mask on. It's the only way I've found to prevent water from getting into my eye area and making me feel even worse.

– Very good – said the doctor trying to remain serious – let's do the tests and find out which component causes the dermatitis. In any case, I guarantee you that you will be able to go back to showering without wearing a mask and snorkel.

The tests revealed that Giulio was not allergic to water at all but to nickel, a metal present in many substances, including shampoos, shower gels and soaps. The solution was simple: a local therapy together with the elimination of all products that contained nickel were sufficient to definitively solve his problem.

Giulio was finally able to start showering again like all human beings. He no longer uses a mask and snorkel, not even for snorkelling when he goes on holiday by the sea.

PRECIOUS PILL N.5

Allergies cause a significant deterioration in the quality of life, significantly influencing the daily activities of those who suffer from them and those who live next to them.

Self-diagnosis and self-prescribed treatment can favour the development of subsequent and different allergies.

It is essential to undergo allergy tests by contacting a specialist.

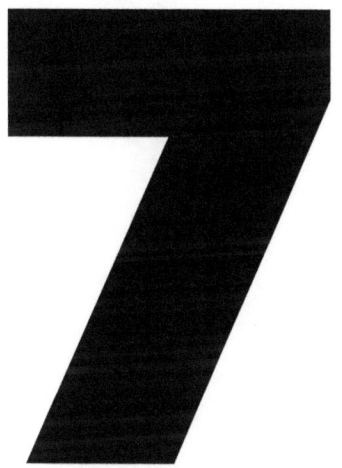

CHAPTER 7 – Case History

COMPANION SNAILS

> Growing up
> he spent his time
> daydreaming about
> his wonderful life
> with furry friends
> without knowing
> that he wouldn't
> be able to make it
> happen.

CHAPTER 7 – CASE HISTORY: COMPANION SNAILS

Basilio had always loved animals and had wished to own one since he was little. Unfortunately, his parents did not agree and so he had never been able to enjoy the company of a dog or a cat.

He thought "when I grow up, I'll get two or maybe three. Yes, maybe a dog and two cats. Or not, maybe there are too many to handle. Let's make a dog and a cat. I'll call them Fuffi and Wolf."

Growing up, he spent his time daydreaming about his wonderful life in the company of furry friends, without knowing that he wouldn't be able to make it happen: an annoying allergy to dust caused him breathing difficulties and forced him to constantly clean every corner of the house to not feel sick or wake up in the middle of the night looking for the inhaler on the bedside table.

He had noticed, in fact, that every time he found himself in the presence of an animal or went to visit someone who owned pets, he struggled to breathe and had to move away before having a full-blown respiratory crisis.

He couldn't give up: his life wouldn't have been the same if he hadn't found his pets at home waiting for him, happy to see him. He absolutely had to find a solution.

One Sunday, while walking in the park near his home, he sat down on a bench to enjoy the morning sun and noticed that a little snail was slowly moving towards him.

He took it in his hand with all the amazement that only an animal lover can feel while observing them. After getting inside its shell to protect itself, the snail slowly came out of its house again and looked out hesitantly as if to taste the danger.

Basilio was fascinated watching the little animal crawl on his palm and thought "Why not? After all, it's an animal too."

Very carefully, so as not to scare his new friend, he returned home, taking it with him.

He entered the kitchen, opened the fridge and took two salad leaves from the stump. He put them in the sink and placed the little snail on top. He went into the bedroom and took a laundry box down from the wardrobe and emptied it onto the bed. He washed it, dried it well and returned to the kitchen with some anxiety. Luckily the snail had moved only a little. Well.

He quickly left the house and returned to the park, where he quickly filled a shopping bag with clods of dirt and grass.

Once back in the house, he rushed to check that the snail hadn't managed to climb up the sink and perhaps end up falling to the floor.

No, luckily it was always there busy nibbling on the salad. Basilio took the box and covered it with grass, then placed the snail in it and chopped more lettuce to feed it.

CHAPTER 7 – CASE HISTORY: COMPANION SNAILS

He finally had an animal too!

"I'll call it Lea" he said to himself and then, addressing the animal directly, he added: "Do you like your new home, Lea? Soon you will have some little friends too."

Then he returned to the park and started looking for other snails to adopt. When he had found a dozen he felt satisfied and took them home.

Every evening when he came home, first thing, he went to check on his little friends and feed them. His desire to have a dog, however, was felt stronger than ever, so he decided to go and visit an allergy specialist to whom he could explain his problems and his wishes.

– I really want an animal, Doctor, but I'm allergic. However, for a year now I have had snails and I have no problems with them: they give me so much joy.

– Let me understand, do you have snails as pets? – asked Doctor Di Rienzo Businco.

– Sure! You should see them doctor, when I come home in the evening, they are so happy to see me that you can see their happiness!

– The snails. They are happy to see you... But how do they do that, do they move their "little horns" quickly? – The doctor said, still with a professional attitude despite the situation.

– As well! And then they rush towards me as soon as they see me.

– They rush... but are you really sure that they are common snails?

Basilio smiled. Then he sighed.

– Doctor, so to speak... Can you see what my love for animals makes me do? Can you help me, please?

– Of course – replied the allergist – when were you diagnosed with allergies to dog and cat hair?

– I never was, but every time I find myself close to an animal, I have a breathing crisis.

– I understand. So, you are not sure if you are allergic...

– I'm definitely allergic to dust, I was diagnosed with it ten years ago.

– Very good. Let's do this: we repeat all the tests, see exactly what causes the crises and then we'll decide what to do.

The tests revealed that Basilio was allergic to dust – as he had long known – but not to animals. The problem lay elsewhere: animals, especially long-haired ones, retain in their fur the dust they collect from the environment. Breathing crises in the presence of pets were always triggered by dust, and not by the dog nor by the cat itself.

The desensitization therapy solved Basilio's problems; as soon as he felt better, he got a dog and a cat, fulfilling his lifelong dream.

However, there was no further news of his snails.

PRECIOUS PILL N.6

Allergies, when left untreated, end up affecting life in both small and big ways.

Not undergoing adequate tests prevents finding a definitive solution to what could turn out to be a reaction to an allergen other than the one independently identified.

Today the solution exists and is available to everyone. Why settling for a life below the standards we wish for when it is possible to solve the problem once and for all?

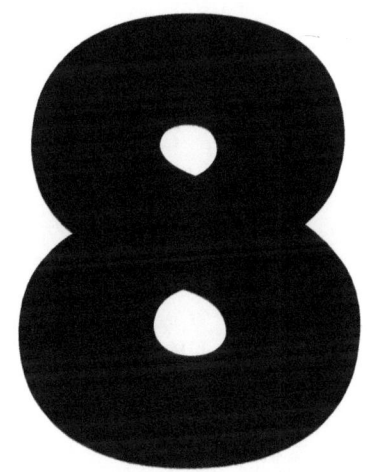

CHAPTER 8

THE DESENSITIZATION THERAPY

> Obviously, the company's quality standard affects its core business, specifically allergies: using cutting-edge technology to produce top-level medicines.

Let's get to the point! What is the desensitization therapy? How is it produced? Is it a new therapy?

History

I am going to start from the beginning, from 1959 when in Haarlem, a town in the Netherlands, a Dutch doctor with an unpronounceable name realized that house dust was responsible for some allergic reactions.

Holed up in a garage, exactly as Steve Jobs did many years later when he created Apple (clearly, garages have a stimulating action on neurons) Dr. Kuijper carries out his experiments on the dust collected at home with a normal vacuum cleaner (can you believe it?), some simple equipment and a lot of ingenuity, pursuing the goal of finding a cure for allergic asthma. He thus laid the foundations for what would become HAL Allergy, today a modern biopharmaceutical company.

In 1965 he produced the first standardized series of allergens for skin tests and the following year he introduced the first extract to fight house dust mites. From this moment on, it was a succession of innovations both in the diagnosis and treatment of allergies in order to improve, optimize and increase the tolerability and effectiveness of the therapy.

A small family

In 1980 HAL Allergy moved to larger and more sophisticated laboratories where the Dutch doctor could better control the synthesis and extracts that were produced. Born as a small "family", the company grows over time, maintaining that attention and care for customers that is not expected from multinationals in the pharmaceutical field: do you understand why I chose to work here?

Integrity, teamwork, responsibility and excellence are the key words that identify the heart of the company and which correspond to my personal values. In 2009 the opening of the new cutting-edge and GMP certified facility in the Bio Science Park of Leiden in the Netherlands led the company to another level, establishing it among the most innovative laboratories.

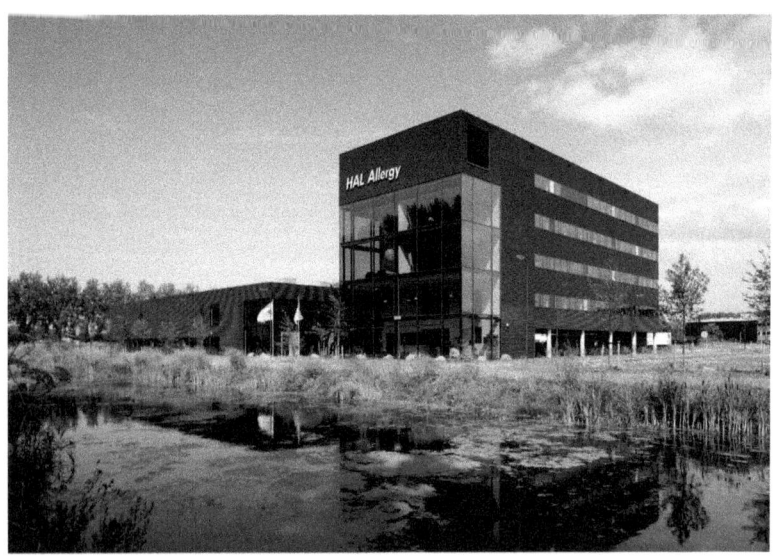

CHAPTER 8 - THE DESENSITIZATION THERAPY

From "The Sorcerer's Apprentice" in the home garage it moved on to "A Space Odyssey": with 3000 m^2 available for production and 2700 m^2 of laboratories and offices, today HAL Allergy represents a safe bet for those suffering from allergic diseases. And there's more! Since the high quality of its technologies is recognised, the company has allocated part of its laboratories to the production of drugs on behalf of other companies and can count the Bill & Melinda Gates Foundation among its first customers, as it chose HAL Allergy to produce HIV drugs to be distributed in developing countries.

Obviously, the company's quality standard affects its core business, specifically allergies: using cutting-edge technology to produce top-level medicines.

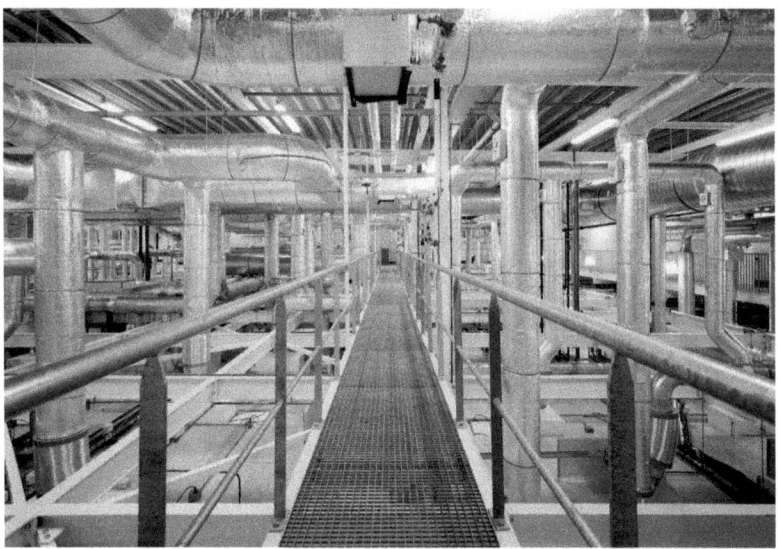

The attention to every single detail, from the purity of the water, to the filtering of the air, which must be free of contaminants, and to the constant temperature of each area of the laboratories, confirms its excellence and makes it look like an ultra-modern spaceship. I can definitely state that science fiction – the one in Star Wars or Star Trek – was inspired by our laboratories! 60% of its employees are researchers because the company's mission is to always discover the best solutions for patients.

In over 60 years of history the company has developed a philosophy of excellence, both for innovation and for the approach of closeness to its interlocutors: in fact, it is not satisfied with developing high quality products, but wishes to be recognized as an important point of reference in the allergology field. For this reason, it always tries to create collaborations and develop paths together with its intorlocutors, in order to grow together.

Interesting, isn't it?

As a mother who had to choose the best treatment for her child, I think it is important to also provide that information that leads to trust in a company and, consequently, in the product it offers, especially because a company is made up of people with their own values and ideals and they are the ones who make the difference.

What is it about exactly? How is the therapy produced, what is inside it, how does it work?

Let's have a deeper look

Nature itself is at the basis of the therapy. This means that the raw material, that is the starting point on the path to the finished product and, therefore, to the therapy, is represented by pollen, epithelia or mites, depending on the type of allergy. This raw material is produced by specialized companies that have production sites in various countries. For these companies, producers of herbs or pollen, it is essential to guarantee the purity and germination capacity of the seed.

This means preparing the soil adequately, locating it away from residential areas and free of heavy metals and pesticides, providing the necessary nutrients to the land, planning sowing and collecting only the best product – the pollen, for example, that has fallen far from the plant no longer fits and is therefore excluded.

Once the raw material has been collected, the "healthy" components are extracted from the pollen or herbs to minimize the allergenic ones through specialized machinery, which are used to extract, eliminate impurities, dry, filter and obtain an intact product as the final phase. This is because pollen and grasses have great biological variability, with ionic strengths and bonding capacities different from each other. It is essential, therefore, to be able to isolate the most homogeneous and pure pollen or grass possible. To get an idea of the amount of work, just think that from a kilo of raw material only one gram of pollen suitable for the production of the desensitization therapy is extracted.

What a surprise, isn't it? Who could imagine how much work lies behind a simple phial of desensitization therapy.

What if the allergen to be produced is that of dust mites?
In this case it is not possible to reproduce the process in natural environments, given the large quantity needed to produce one gram of allergen. Also in this case, very strict measures are complied with as far as the cultivation medium is concerned, which must have specific climatic conditions and provide the nourishment necessary for growth and procreation.

Obviously, in this case as well purification processes are carried out to eliminate all foreign substances and obtain the purest base for the production of the therapy.

In all cases, whether plants or animals, after the first purification and quality control phase, the raw material must undergo a second purification phase which takes place in the laboratories of the companies which produce the desensitization therapies.

Let's play with the chemistry set

The allergens, therefore, or rather the proteic part causing the allergy, is extracted from the raw material (the one obtained after the first purification) through aqueous solutions with a constant pH and are filtered to obtain homogeneous glycoproteins, all the same, eliminating the pigments that can cause irritative reactions.

At this point it is necessary to measure the strength, the intensity of the allergens, through specific tests: prick tests, intradermal and rast.

In all three cases, the tests are used to validate the intensity of the allergens because the standardization requires that each company complies with the principles of homogeneity, reproducibility and allergic intensity of its products. The allergens tested must correspond to the "samples" which are present in the company: in short, each batch produced must have the same characteristics.

Is that all? No. Here we are halfway through the process: we have obtained an intermediate product between raw material and drug, which must be adapted to be administered to patients.

In the case of sublingual therapy, HAL Allergy adds *glycerol, peppermint* and other excipients to the intermediate product, thus obtaining drops to be placed under the tongue.

If, instead, *aluminium hydroxide* and *glutaraldehyde* are added to the intermediate product, subcutaneous therapy is produced.

To make it clear – I understand that these are difficult terms for those who have never heard of them – *aluminium hydroxide* is a stabilizer – it is used to keep the solution stable – and is used in microscopic doses, while *glutaraldehyde* is a kind of carrier or vector, which allows side effects to be reduced while keeping the effectiveness of the therapy constant.

HAL Allergy uses *glutaraldehyde*, a substance that modifies the original structure of the allergen into another called *allergoid*, where the allergen is masked – and since it is not recognized by the immune system, it does not activate the defensive reaction – but inside the body it can reach the place where it must act – taking off its mask, like Zorro, in short – without causing side effects.

At this point in the procedure, a group of 19 analysts carries out tests on each batch of product, for a total of 21,000 tests per year, which help verify every aspect: the colour, the presence of precipitation, the allergenic power, the underwater material and so on, in order to guarantee the high quality standard which is the flag of the company itself.

Not yet satisfied, HAL Allergy, obsessed as it is with the concept of high quality, has also activated the voluntary process of "who inspects the inspector?" and therefore after ONLY 21,000 tests have been performed by the analysts, the samples of each batch are sent to the Paul-Ehrlich-Institut, the equivalent of AIFA (Italian Medicines Agency) for further control.

The approval from the certifying body allows the product to be placed on the market and followed up to the end user, who is the patient.

It is important to me to explain all this because neither the patients nor the doctors often know how much work goes into it and the value that a phial of product has.

The mechanism of action of the desensitization therapy

How exactly does the therapy work? How does it work?

Every living being on Earth, plant or animal, is made up of various substances, including proteins, without which there is no life.

Some of them, however, can be, for no specific reason, particularly annoying for human beings. That is, the immune system recognizes them as dangerous for the body and activates an immediate defence which shows itself through sneezing, coughing, tearing or bronchospasm.

The desensitization therapy aims at ensuring that the immune system learns to get to know these substances/allergens, preventing those violent reactions from triggering. The therapy works through the introduction of very small quantities of those same allergens at regular intervals into the individual, to give our immune system time to identify them if not as friends at least as acquaintances.

The journey of the allergen

Imagine the scene: whether it is drops or subcutaneous therapy, the allergens that cause such disabling symptoms are introduced into the body.

The small quantities of allergens are like foreigners starting a journey to discover a new country.

They travel in very small groups, to better integrate with the environment they will encounter. When they arrive, they find a border to cross to gain access. The guardian (the immune system) is watchful, suspicious, observes them, controls them, lets them in little by little and at regular intervals.

At the same time, other travellers arrive (always the same allergens) who join the first ones, waiting to meet again. Our guardian (always the immune system), which is conscientious, waits a little longer but in the meantime has already seen that the new arrivals are the same as the first, they have the same smell, appearance and characteristics. In other words, they are familiar to him, he knows that maybe they are a little loud but not bad and from this moment on he welcomes them without any more problems.

They might be the allergenic proteins deriving from the epithelium of our beloved cat or grandma's lively poodle.

Or they are the widespread dust mites: they cannot be seen, they cannot be heard, they do not bite, they do not sting but they are with us by the millions.

They are among the oldest living beings on earth and, me being a palaeontologist, they should fascinate me, but I get itchy just saying their name. They can grow in different environments: those responsible for asthma, for example, are those of house dust which have their habitat in the domestic environment.

Man succumbs not only to mites but also to the stings of bees and wasps, the so-called Hymenoptera family. Even in this case, the desensitization therapy, it must be said, can change your life, or rather, saves it. The sting of these insects, in fact, can cause an anaphylactic shock and the death of the patient.

Password: Quality

All this seems to be ignored by the patient or rather underestimated. Yet, the desensitization therapy which, as already mentioned, is the only one recognized by the World Health Organization as a therapy that cures the cause, is a truly effective therapy. At HAL Allergy we not only guarantee effectiveness, but as mentioned, quality.

The quality, of the highest level, is controlled throughout the production chain, from the choice of land, to the laboratories, tests, production, up to distribution, another point of pride for the company: each phial is "customised" – term which means studied and adapted to the patient in the same way as a tailored suit: the therapy is tailor-made, therefore, based on the specialist's request for that patient, inserted in a box with the patient's name and delivered directly to the patient's home.

We can talk about precision or personalized medicine, because these are absolutely not one-size-fits-all over-the-counter drugs.

Each transport phase is controlled like everything else and

guaranteed by the cold chain which keeps the product at a constant temperature until it reaches the patient's hands.

The Client Service

This is what we call "placing the patient at the centre" of the activity and not considering him just like an end customer: every step is optimized to provide our client with the maximum in terms of quality, safety and effectiveness.

This last aspect is essential for us and for this reason we have a Client Service system available to our patients.

From the moment the patient sends the prescription, we are at their disposal for the entire duration of the therapy, helping them solve any problem or provide them with the information they need.

This is what happened, for example, during the Covid-19 pandemic: patients constantly called to find out if they could follow the therapy, what interaction there could be between the therapy and the vaccine or the virus, and what to do in their specific case and according to the situation they were experiencing.

We are deeply persuaded – and our actions prove it – that patient support should not be limited to providing a drug, but goes far beyond: we want to be a point of reference to turn to in order to fully support the patient on the path to a better quality of life.

CHAPTER 8 - THE DESENSITIZATION THERAPY

We guarantee presence and collaboration to also help patients to be constant and not to quit the therapy before the end of three years, the time necessary to achieve a complete desensitization.

The WhatsApp chat is active 24 hours a day and was created to tell the patient *"Speak, I'm listening"*, something that rarely happens in everyday life.

We are always in a hurry and even specialists are reluctant to give more attention than what is strictly necessary to their patients, because time is a fundamental resource.

For us, however, dedicating time to patients is an integral part of our philosophy and our way of saying *"I care about you"*.

During the Covid period, we received a disproportionate number of calls, emails and WhatsApp messages from patients, often asking us questions that went beyond allergies. Many of them wanted to be reassured, others wanted confirmation, many wanted to be sure that their behaviour was the right one.

We didn't give any indications that weren't our responsibility, of course, but we were able to calm and reassure everyone by offering a listening ear and dedicated time. Experience has shown us that being truly at the service of the patient makes the difference, because each of them doesn't just need drugs: they want to be accompanied on the recovery journey knowing that there is someone who will answer them if necessary.

HAL Allergy Italy for Social issues

Attention to the patient, it is now more than clear, is our mantra, but not only: "Good thoughts, good words, good actions" and HAL Allergy Italia is a company that pays attention to social issues, a fundamental ethical value. This means feeling deeply involved in what happens, be present.

For this reason, during the first wave of the pandemic, the Italian office conceived and activated, in collaboration with Avalon Counselling, the totally free *Prima Linea* [Front Line– TN] project, a counselling service, started in Lombardy and then extended to the whole Italian territory, which everyone could turn to – healthcare workers, doctors, nurses, porters... – in a specific time slot to meet a counsellor and talk in serenity and confidentiality about what they were experiencing. We wanted to be close to all the operators

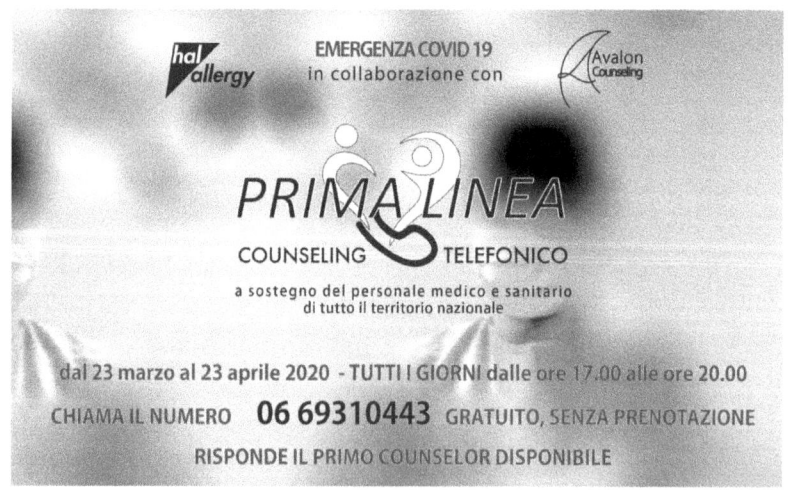

CHAPTER 8 - THE DESENSITIZATION THERAPY

who found themselves, overnight, managing a situation they knew nothing about but which was claiming victims in rapid succession. *Prima Linea* was really a success and we are proud of it.

Beauty will save us! This is why we support ART and we did so in 2020 by promoting the issuing of the photographic book "PANDEMIC ART" by Fabrizio Gatta with the aim of starting again from culture. Photographic follies that tell, through the photographer's lens and with a metaphor, the impact that the pandemic has had on every sector of society.

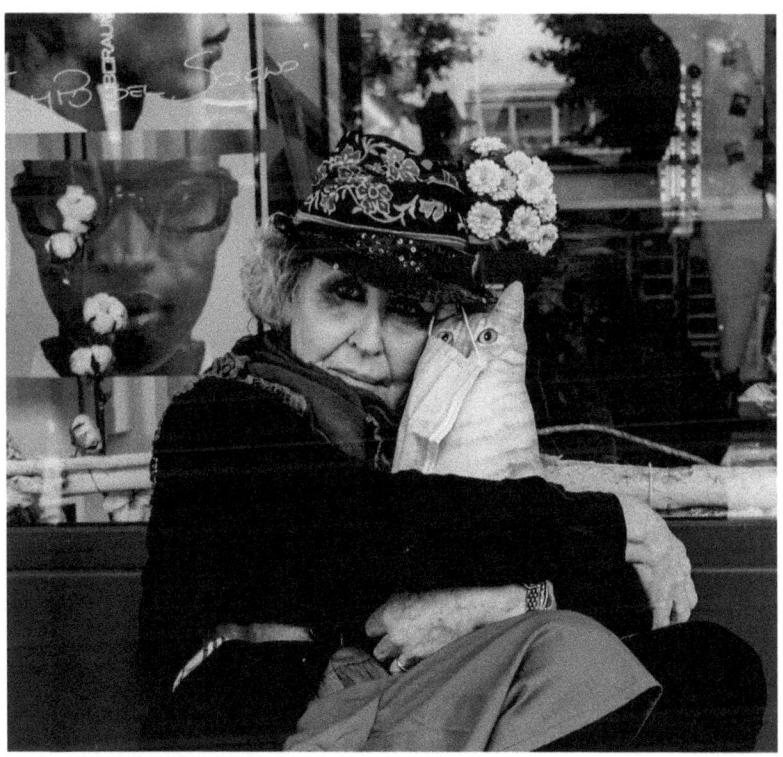

Going further, this is my vision and in 2021 we started funding a scholarship at the Niko Romito Academy of Haute Cuisine, because we believe that nutrition contributes to a healthy life and the general well-being of people and we share the same philosophy of the multi-starred chef based on culture and training.

Health and food go hand in hand, and it is essential for a future chef to understand the differences between intolerances and allergies. Hence the focus, included in the Academy's program, on food allergies. The latest activity launched at HAL Allergy Italia are monthly webinars on the Zoom platform, which everyone can access for free by booking their place.

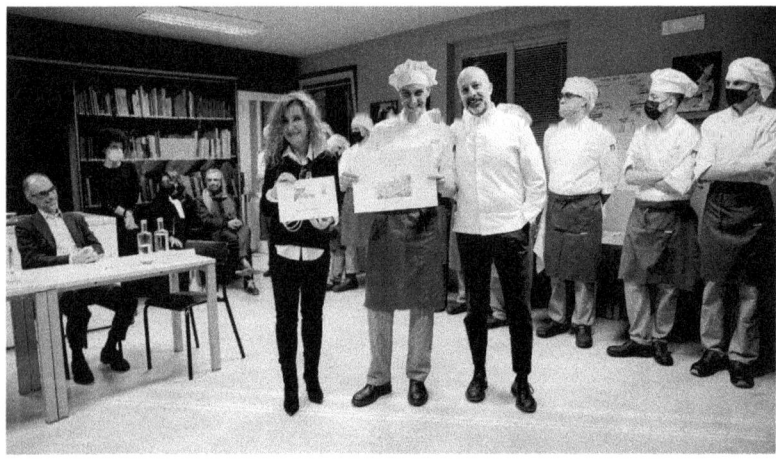

These are meetings on different topics – not only on allergies and their management – but on topics that can affect daily life: the

CHAPTER 8 - THE DESENSITIZATION THERAPY

creams we use, the foods we eat, or how to handle the relationship with an allergic child.

To get information on the agenda of the events that will take place the upcoming months, simply send an email to info@halallergy.it writing "calendar of event dates" in the object and, once you have found what is of your interest, apply to participate.

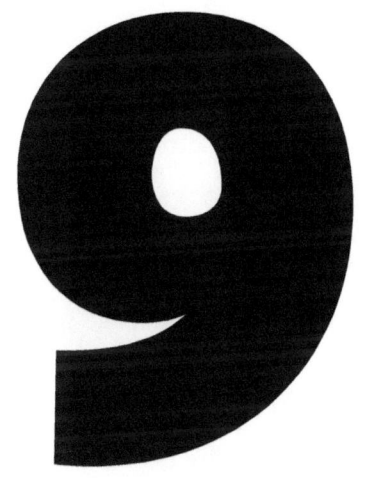

CHAPTER 9

THE NHS AND THE DESENSITIZATION THERAPIES: WHO PAYS FOR THEM? COST OR VALUE?

> I still remember that day and the quick decision taken in line with our patient-oriented philosophy: we kept the same cost for patients in order to guarantee continuity of therapy, even if this meant a net loss for the company.

CHAPTER 9 - THE NHS AND THE DESENSITIZATION THERAPIES: WHO PAYS FOR THEM? COST OR VALUE?

At the end of this book, a short chapter dedicated to costs could not be missing, as it is in our interest to inform patients about every aspect of the desensitization therapy. According to Article 32 of the Italian Constitution, in Italy there should be uniformity of services provided to citizens and prices, because everyone has the same right to health; however, the actual situation is very different.

With the transfer of power in the health field from the central government to the regions – which have become responsible for the health service in their territory – diversified approaches have been observed, uniformity has been lost and discordant choices have been made also as far as costs are concerned. This means that depending on the region in which the patient lives, the cost of the drug changes.

The desensitization therapies, which have been on the market for 30 years, are regulated by Article 5 of Ministerial Decree 219 of 2006, which establishes that the so-called *Name-Patient* therapies, that is, nominal therapies – tailor-made for a person – are not sold in pharmacies but ordered directly from pharmaceutical companies through a specialist's prescription.

The pharmaceutical company produces the drug *ad personam* with the patient's name and sends it to their home. Since a regulatory process different from the traditional one is used – and this derives from the fact that the therapy is customizable and not identical for everyone – its reimbursement by the NHS is not contemplated. In other words, the Government does not reimburse part of the cost of the drug as it would for other products. In this scenario, some regions have decided to co-participate totally or partially in the cost of the therapy.

The uneven Italian situation

Lombardy, to name one, supports the costs through a resolution issued several years ago that establishes the number of annual phials that can be reimbursed between seasonal and so-called "perennial" therapies. Piedmont has a different organization: it has created an allergy network of specialists who in this region are the only ones who can prescribe a desensitization therapy. Here, the costs are supported half by the region and half by the patient.

In both cases – in Piedmont and Lombardy – the product is supplied by the Hospital Pharmacy, whose supply comes from a regional tender or a framework agreement.

In a few words, the cost of the product is never the cost to the public – that is, what the patient pays in full in another region – but arises from the tender procedure and is, therefore, significantly lower than the price for the private individual and changes with each new tender.

Puglia has adopted the partial reimbursement strategy based on ISEE income [Indicator of the Equivalent Economic Situation – TN] and until a few years ago Sicily also reimbursed the therapy indirectly: the patient purchased it and the region reimbursed it. Then, due to the mandatory temporary external administration of the region and the cost recovery plan, the reimbursement was cancelled.

I still remember that day and the quick decision taken in line with our patient-oriented philosophy: we kept the same cost for patients in order to guarantee continuity of therapy, even if this meant a net loss for the company.

For the rest of the Italian territory, the reimbursement map is patchy: some regions offer it and others don't. For instance, there are some Local Health Authorities that reimburse the product autonomously, even if the region does not do so, as in the case of Piacenza.

In conclusion, with all due respect to article 32, there are actually first-class and second-class patients, and this depends only on the region in which you live.

What are these costs, anyway?

Let's monetize

Even though the same drug can vary in price from one pharmaceutical company to another, we can say, in general, that for a patient who has to pay privately for the product, the costs amount to around €500 per year for the injectable therapy and €700 for the sublingual one, with some exceptions that can reach around €1000 per year.

Although it corresponds to less than the cost of a coffee a day, and certainly less than what is spent in a lifetime on antihistamines, cortisone and beta-blockers, it is, however, a significant amount that should be reimbursed by the government at least in part.

HAL Allergy is working in order to raise awareness in the regions on this issue and ensure that they reimburse at least part of the cost of the product.

Recently the Lazio region approved a motion and could be among the regions that support this therapy.

What is the situation in the rest of Europe?

In the rest of Europe the situation is completely different and diversified. The greatest use is in Germany, which certainly represents the largest market. The desensitization therapy is fully reimbursed and the difference with Italy is the greater use of the subcutaneous therapy compared to the sublingual therapy.

In Spain the therapy is also reimbursed but 50%, like in Piedmont and here too there is a preference for the injectable therapy.

Reimbursements are also offered in Poland, Austria and the Netherlands. In short, the use of the desensitization therapy is certainly important in Europe.

Value not cost

Back to Italy – and to the cost of the therapy for the patient – I would like to focus on one last point: the difference between cost and value, which is not just a difference in meaning.

Everyone is used to talking about costs, about how much money they have to spend in order to get anything, in this specific case, to benefit from a desensitization therapy. However, we often tend to be a bit superficial.

When we talk about the cost of therapy we should consider the VALUE of the therapy, which is represented by the sum of all the work, research, quality, study and time dedicated to it and which I have already mentioned above; we should not forget the fact that today's products are not those of 30 years ago, precisely because we continue to improve them thanks to scientific research: this is the real value of the desensitization therapy that goes far beyond the purchase cost.

CHAPTER 10

WHAT IF THE LITTLE PRINCE HAD BEEN ALLERGIC?

> When my son was little, I used to read it to him all the time and I remember thinking every time, "If the little prince had been allergic, he wouldn't have been able to have all the experiences he talks about in the book and he wouldn't have had a life full of emotions.

CHAPTER 10 – WHAT IF THE LITTLE PRINCE HAD BEEN ALLERGIC?

I have always loved Antoine de Saint-Exupéry's masterpiece, The Little Prince, because it is a little book that can speak to everyone's hearts, even those who are a little more "grown up" like me. It is one of the most read books in the world because it speaks in a simple way about love, friendship and the meaning of life. When my son was little, I used to read it to him and I remember that every time I thought: "if the little prince had been allergic he would not have been able to have all the experiences he talks about in the book and he would not have had a life full of emotions".

The next thought was to hope that my little prince would get better and be able to enjoy everything in the same way. At that point my son Simone, who has always been an intelligent child, seeing the look of a heartbroken mother in my eyes, addressed me with the words from the book "Adults never understand anything by themselves and it's a bore that children are always eternally forced to explain things to them" making me burst out laughing heartily.

The book tells the story of this little prince, a boy, who meets an aviator in the Sahara desert who has crashed his plane. The boy tells his new friend that he is the prince and the only inhabitant of an asteroid and that he is visiting the planet Earth. Where he lives there are three volcanoes, which he takes care of by sweeping their chimneys every week, a rose – the dearest thing in the world to him – and many baobab trees. The reason for his journey is to find a sheep that will eat from the trees to prevent them from suffocating the planet.

NO MORE TISSUES SABRINA DE FEDERICIS

During his earthly adventure, the Little Prince – whose name we never learn – meets a series of characters and some animals: he becomes friends with a fox who wants to be tamed and a snake which bites him, allowing him to return to his asteroid. Now I wonder: what if the Little Prince had really been allergic? First of all, he could not have lived alone in the middle of a wild nature: he would not have lasted a week without a hospital, medicines and someone to take care of him!

What if he had been allergic to some plants? His best friend in the book is a rose, whose perfume he could not smell, nor could he sit next to it to talk to it without starting to sneeze heavily! What if the baobabs had caused him an allergic reaction? That poor child would have suffered from allergic rhinitis constantly. On his planet there were also three volcanoes: if he had been allergic to a substance contained in the magma or lava, he would not have been able to take care of them for fear of getting close.

The same goes for animals: what would have happened if he had been allergic to the fox fur? The Little Prince would have missed the opportunity to find a new friend in the animal. Finally, what if he had been allergic to snake venom? There is only one answer: the Little Prince would no longer exist. I took this book as an example because even in a children's story – and The Little Prince is much more – there are situations and characters that represent insurmountable problems for an allergic person.

A child who suffers from allergies runs the risk of missing out on many adventures and giving up friends, pets, and runs in the nature, if he is not properly cared for. The same goes for adults: for fear of getting sick, knowing that they cannot control the external environment – be it a restaurant, a friend's house, or a green lawn – they end up shutting themselves at home and giving up socializing. Although The Little Prince does not talk about allergies, a sentence in the book explains this concept perfectly:

"It is madness to hate all roses because one thorn pricked you, to abandon all dreams because one of them didn't come true, to give up on all attempts because one failed. It is madness to condemn all friendships because one betrayed you, to not believe in any love just because one of them was unfaithful, to throw away all the possibilities of being happy just because something didn't go right. There will always be another opportunity, another friendship, another love, a new strength. For every ending there is a new beginning."

For my son – and for me as the mother of an allergy sufferer – the new beginning was precisely discovering that we didn't have to settle for trying to block the symptoms but could solve the problem at the root once and for all, because as the Little Prince says:

"Men grow 5000 roses in the same garden and do not find what they are looking for. And yet what they are looking for could be found in a single rose or in a little water".

Writing this book was a truly special moment in my life at an equally peculiar historical moment.

" Writing this book was a truly special moment in my life at an equally special time in history.

CONCLUSIONS

By putting down on paper my experience as a mother of an allergic child and the different situations that one is called upon to manage at various times, I truly hope to have opened a window of knowledge as well as of hope to all allergic patients who experience this pathology as a misfortune that has occurred in their lives.

You have red hair, she has two-tone eyes, I have allergies! Oh, cruel fate that in the middle of a kiss makes me sneeze, or in a moment of pathos makes my nose itch and me cough in the silence of a church. Telling the story of the desensitization therapy – the only therapy capable of curing the cause of the allergy and not the symptom – and how it is produced, has allowed me to satisfy that need for sharing that I have felt for some time.

Today a cure exists – the desensitization therapy – and it can definitively solve the problem by freeing you from the symptoms and giving you back the joy of living, taking a walk in the park, playing with a pet, smelling the scent of a flower.

As you have learned, the desensitization therapy is not well known because it requires a great deal of commitment on your part: to be constant and to not give up for three years, to give the allergen enough time to communicate with the immune system. Unfortunately, patients often stop it early, as soon as they see an improvement, without obtaining the long-lasting results that the therapy guarantees. Furthermore, in some Italian regions the treatment is not supported by the National Health System, thus persuading some of those who learn about it to take the decision not to follow it.

As I explained in chapter 7, however, if you do your math carefully you will realize that not only is the annual cost less than that of a coffee a day, but also that it is significantly lower than the cost of the drugs that you are forced to take for life without ever solving the problem.

My desire is to provide you with the tools to make a conscious choice and decide whether you prefer to continue taking antihistamines and cortisone or stop taking any drug in three years.

I would like to thank Dr. Andrea Di Rienzo Businco for his tireless work, for the case histories he allowed me to include in this book, embracing its playful spirit.

The allergist, often an underestimated professional, is the only one capable of "seeing" the symptoms as a whole, even when they concern different districts, and proposing a therapy built around the patient as in a high fashion tailoring.

CONCLUSIONS

It is very important to consult an allergist because with their help you can heal and leave behind discomfort, disorders and sacrifices.

I chose this way of telling the story because, as the mother of an allergic child, I know how difficult it can be to live with allergies, both for those who suffer from them as well as for those around them or, as unfortunately happens, for those who have to rush to the hospital in the middle of the night for a breathing crisis. Above all, driven by the awareness, after having spoken to and listened to many allergic patients, of the great loneliness that one feels in managing a pathology classified as "not very important" or, otherwise said, "secondary" only because it does not have the mortality rate of a cardiac or oncological pathology.

Not deadly, not so frequently at least, but certainly debilitating for the quality of life of those who experience it firsthand. Even more insidious, perhaps, because it limits the most important thing we have, "sociality": no parks, no gardens, no soccer games, no running in the woods or picnics on the grass; no dogs, no cats, no curtains, and so on, a series of Nothings. And it is for this Nothing that I wanted to write the book: to tell everyone that this Nothing can transform into an EVERYTHING because there has been, for some time, a curative therapy for allergies from inhalants.

The Therapy that, one could say, allows you to breathe again, to regain the playing field, to reduce or stop taking antihistamines, cortisone and to finally forget about the Tissues.

With "No more tissues" I tried to provide pure information, bringing to the attention of the allergy sufferers that healing is possible, indeed it is necessary, because it is only a question of choice.

Choose, then, to do it.

GLOSSARY

AIFA: Italian Medicines Agency

Allergy: Exaggerated reactivity (hyperergy) acquired by the organism towards a particular substance (allergen) that has previously sensitized it.

Allergen: In medicine, any substance capable of causing a state of allergy.

Allergoid: allergens modified and optimized in their structure.

Antihistamine: Drug that opposes the action of histamine, used in the symptomatology of allergic diseases.

Cortisone: anti-inflammatory and immunosuppressive drugs, with a structure similar to endogenous corticosteroids.

Excipients: in pharmaceuticals, a pharmacologically inert substance with little chemical reactivity that gives a medicinal preparation the necessary shape, consistency, dilution and other chemical-physical characteristics, acting above all as a vehicle for the active substances.

Ionic forces: quantities used to express the intensity of the electric field of an electrolytic solution.

Glycerol: organic compound in whose structure there are three Hydroxy groups.

Glycoproteins: proteins to whose peptide chain an oligosaccharide chain is linked.

Glutaraldehyde: almost colourless liquid with a pungent odour.

GMP: Good Manufacturing Practices.

Aluminum hydroxide: A substance used as a stabilizer to prevent chemical reactions within the product.

Intradermal: A skin test to determine if a patient is allergic. Allergens are injected under the patient's skin.

Hymenoptera: an order of insects that includes over 120,000 species spread throughout the world.

Paul-Ehrlich-Institut: Agency of the German Ministry of Health. Equivalent of AIFA.

GLOSSARY

Prick Test: a diagnostic test used to identify the causes of a respiratory or food allergy. It is performed by lightly pricking the skin with a special lancet and applying a drop of allergen to the skin of the forearm.

Rast: a type of blood test aimed at identifying possible allergens responsible for allergies in humans.

Standardization: A process carried out using reference preparations consisting of controlled extracts against which each new production batch is compared.

Desensitization therapy: a therapy for allergic pathology that consists of the administration of increasing doses of an extract that contains the substance that causes the allergy.

AFTERWORD
BY PAOLO CIANI

BREATHING IS A FUNDAMENTAL RIGHT

The book you are about to read was written two years ago and is the story of a therapy that cures respiratory allergies caused by inhalant allergens and is not satisfied with numbing the symptoms. A clear, linear story that communicates in a simple way how the person with allergies is not destined to be sick for life but can educate their immune system to come into relation with natural substances that, for some strange reason, it considers as foreign bodies to defend itself from.

I was glad to write the afterword as requested by the author. I had had the opportunity months before meeting Sabrina to come into contact with the so little considered problem of respiratory allergies. In our meetings I had the chance to fully understand the situation, to recognise how the allergic population was alone in facing their pathology and also in bearing the cost of the therapy that "cures" the allergy. Indeed, the disparity of treatment in the dispensation of this therapy in the different Italian regions made me understand how the distance between the National Health System and the people with pathologies is increasingly widening. Not only that, the disparities in treatment between citizens are growing depending on whether they live in Lombardy or Lazio and this, in our opinion, is not acceptable.

I had the chance to appreciate Sabrina's ethics and her dedication to social causes, which is why I accepted to write the afterword of the book; I truly consider *Butta Via i Fazzoletti* [No More Tissues – TN] a book with a social purpose that aims not only to communicate the existence of a "curative" therapy for allergies, but also to raise awareness among political institutions towards a profound discomfort that undermines the quality of life of the person with allergies and of the entire family unit that surrounds them.

As representatives of Demos we are very concerned by the citizens' health and we therefore promote a policy of inclusion aimed at overcoming the disparities in the delivery of health services, of which the desensitization therapy is proof. As I said in the afterword, some time ago I promoted a motion in the Lazio Region in order to start a process of joint participation of the Region itself in the cost of the therapy, a process that I am attentively following up. In the meantime, however, my role has changed and from regional Councillor today I am a Demos Deputy in the Chamber of Deputies. A role that even more requires me to give voice to those minorities that are not considered either because they are too small or because they are neglected by society or, as in the case of people with allergies, because the pathology is underestimated and can be quickly fixed with the use of antihistamines and cortisone. And this despite the fact that this pathology affects 12 million people in Italy and 1 million and two hundred thousand people in the Lazio region. For this reason, I have promoted an interparliamentary group that works on drafting a **PARLIAMENTARY PACT ON RESPIRATORY ALLERGIES**, which could engage the Government, Parliament, Regions and all political forces so that this pathology finds a relevant place in the political, governmental and parliamentary agenda. A 10-point parliamentary pact was therefore prepared, on the basis of which I presented an interpellation that will be discussed in Parliament. I am truly happy with the adhesion of my colleagues to this intergroup, as well as with the response of the scientific societies in the sector, patient associations, "Cittadinanza Attiva" and many others.

The work of these months has also allowed us to draft the First **MANIFESTO** of the rights of people with allergies. I believe it represents an extremely important document that highlights the need to expand the territorial network of specialists in order to guarantee easy accessibility to medical visits, as well as knowledge of the problems inherent to allergies. Not only that, it represents the first official document dedicated to people with respiratory allergies. A "Magna Carta" to protect these silent people who are often resigned to a fate that they consider, erroneously, inevitable.
I am truly grateful to Sabrina for making me aware of this issue, for caring about people's well-being and for wanting to share her

personal experience as a mother of a child - now a young man - who suffered from allergies, and as a professional in the sector with a significant expertise. It will be my concern, in the coming months, to continue this path that is so important for so many millions of people.

Paolo Ciani

Regional Councillor
President of the Special Commission for the COVID-19 emergency
Vice President of the 7th Commission – Health, social policies, social and health integration, welfare
Member of the 10th Commission – Urban planning, housing policies, waste
Member of the Special Commission on area plans for affordable and popular housing in the Region
Member of the 13th Commission – Transparency and advertising Capitoline Assembly
Member of the 5th Commission – Social and Health Policies
7th Commission – Heritage and Housing Policies
12th Commission – Tourism, Fashion and International Relations

AFTERWORD
BY GIANFRANCO FORTUNATO

It was my wedding anniversary, October 16th, 2016. I have never forgotten that day. I was in the countryside, doing some cleaning under the olive trees, when I must have hit a wasp nest with the lawnmower. Suddenly I felt a sharp pain in the back of my neck: I had been stung right on the vein. I had already been stung by various insects during my walks in the woods in search of wild asparagus and I had never had any problems.

That time, however, things were different, and I noticed it immediately: a strong burning sensation in my chest and my vision starting to blur made me leave everything to run to my car and rush to the nearest hospital which was, luckily, only three kilometres away.

I was halfway there when I started having trouble breathing, and shortly after, while I was running to get to the emergency room, I also had a small accident when I ended up off the road. It was thanks to a boy who stopped to help me, and to whom I just had time to tell that I had been stung by a bee or a wasp, if I'm still alive. I regained consciousness while the doctors were about to intubate me.

NO MORE TISSUES   SABRINA DE FEDERICIS

I was hospitalized for three days on an IV drip and during that forced stay, partly because of some memories and partly from the stories told by the boy who had helped me, I discovered that I had arrived at the hospital already cyanotic and that it had also been necessary to administer adrenaline to me.

In the months that followed, I had several visits and prick tests that confirmed a very strong allergy to wasps and then, in the hospital, I began an intravenous therapy with which I was infused with small doses of wasp venom. Obviously, everything took place in a protected environment (hospital) so that the doctors could be able to intervene in case of a new shock.

Today, I have been undergoing this desensitization therapy for seven years and even though I have been stung four more times, I haven't had any more serious reactions. From this personal experience of mine, the Molise Allergy Patients Association was born, which has the aim of supporting in various ways all those who fight with this pathology, too often underestimated.

This is the reason why, when Sabrina asked me to write the afterword to this book, I was glad: what better testimony than the story of a personal experience – how allergies not only drastically undermine the quality of life of those who suffer from them and their loved ones but can even lead to death.

The desensitization therapy, in the case of wasp stings, is a lifesaver: you need patience, perseverance and time but it allows you to return to leading a normal life. This is the wish I make for all of you, to be able to return to living normally in the Nature that surrounds us.

Gianfranco Fortunato

President APAM – Molise Allergy Patients Association.

THANK YOU FOR READING THIS FAR!

If you have read this far, there are three, or rather four, cases:

- you are an allergic person;
- you are a relative of an allergic person;
- you are a doctor who has allergic patients;
- you want to know more about the risks that arise from allergies.

Whatever the reason that pushed you to read my book to the end, I want to thank you, for me it is very important to receive your feedback and to know if this work of mine has been useful to you, if the information you have found on these pages has helped to clarify the foggy world of allergies and available treatments.

For this reason, I ask you to leave me feedback on Amazon, I will be truly grateful.

I remind you that for any curiosity, doubt, request for information, you can contact me by writing to this email address: info@halallergy.it

If you want to receive the chart to evaluate if you are a potential allergy sufferer, you can text me on WhatsApp: 0039 3491446699
I wish you a life in which you can breathe deeply and... without tissues!

www.buttaviaifazzoletti.it

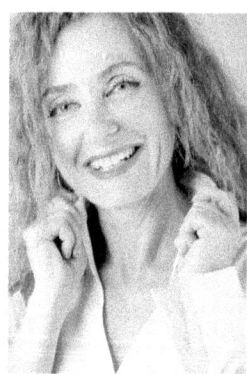

ACKNOWLEDGEMENTS

The strength of the Individual can never equal the strength of the Group and, in this case, the group was represented by all those who, in some way, supported this idea, dedicated their time to it and, above all, have always cheered for me.

First of all my son Simone, a source of inspiration not only for the book but for life itself. From him I continue to receive important life lessons.

My partner Valerio who sees my madness as normal. My colleagues at HAL Allergy, including Roberta Mariotti with her thousand resources and Giuseppe Bonanno, , with his preparation and deep knowledge of the desensitization therapy, supervised the most technical part.

A special thanks to Dr. Andrea Di Rienzo Businco, for giving us pieces of his experience with patients, for his willingness to follow me in this adventure and for his friendship.

My gratitude goes to Paolo Ciani, Lazio Regional Councillor, President of the Special Commission for the COVID-19 emergency, Vice President of the 7th Commission – Health, social policies, social and health integration, welfare, for the afterword but above all for the concrete political commitment aimed at obtaining a co-participation of the Lazio region in the desensitization therapy.

A further thank you to the President of the Molise Patients Association, Gianfranco Fortunato, for his testimony and for all the work he is doing, together with lawyer Ciarniello, in the Molise region for the reimbursement of the aforementioned therapy.

To the Niko Romito Academy of Haute Cuisine, for having included in the training course a day dedicated to the world of allergies, understanding its cultural importance.

To Fabrizio Gatta, a great photographer and above all a great friend with whom I have shared many work experiences.

A special and unique thanks to Zuleika Fusco, life teacher, relationship counsellor, from whom I learned so much and who taught me to be who I am. With her I had the honour of developing the social project "Prima Linea" [Front Line – TN].

Finally I want to thank *Libri d'Impresa* for helping "No More Tissues" to become the magnificent reality of an e-book and also of paper and ink, upon request.

ACKNOWLEDGEMENTS

It was extraordinary to have found so many people ready to share my same enthusiasm and to support me and tolerate me in this small enterprise.

All this was possible only thanks to each of you.

BIOGRAPHY

Sabrina de Federicis lives and works in Rome as Country Manager of the pharmaceutical company HAL Allergy. Although she works in the pharmaceutical industry, she has always cultivated other interests.

She is a Relationship Counsellor with a focus on Communication Media. She has a degree in the scientific field with a specialization in Human Palaeontology. She is a scientific communicator and an expert in creating effective relationships, developing brand identity, planning business, and developing creative solutions.

"No More Tissues" is her first book.

APPENDIX

MANIFESTO OF THE RIGHTS AND DUTIES OF PERSONS WITH RESPIRATORY ALLERGIES

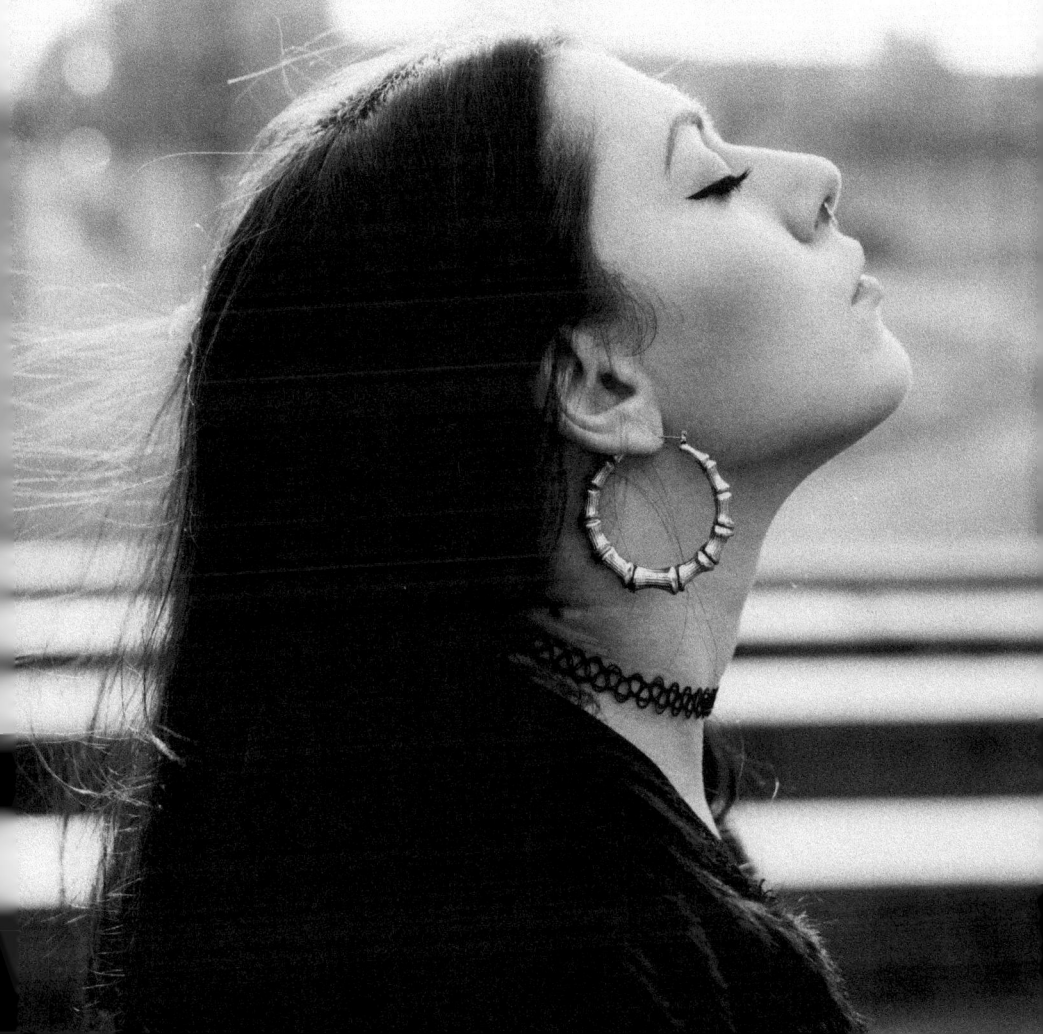

FOREWORD

Respiratory allergies represent a global problem and entail a significant social and economic burden to national health systems;

According to the World Health Organization and data in the literature, approximately 350 million people worldwide suffer from diseases related to respiratory allergies, such as rhinitis and bronchial asthma;

The aforementioned diseases are chronic and heavily influence the quality of life of people with major social, economic and clinical implications;

The appearance and recurrence of symptoms (especially cough and breathing difficulty) require a demanding handling, with regular, urgent specialist visits and even hospitalizations for the management of the most severe cases;

According to the US Center for Disease Control and Prevention (CDC), children with respiratory allergies miss twice as many days of school as their peers;

In Italy, approximately 10% of children under 14 suffer from asthma and 80% of them are allergic;

Respiratory allergies are the cause of asthma in 80% of cases and it is therefore essential to act on their prevention;

In order to prevent respiratory diseases, an essential element is represented by the observation, in the first years of life, of the origin of numerous chronic lung diseases in adults, including asthma, which unfortunately record still worrying morbidity and mortality rates;

The US National Institute of Health has identified the hypothesis that the increase in the level of hygiene and exposure to pollutants, typical of the most advanced societies in the world, influences the immune response by promoting allergic sensitization;

Furthermore, in addition to the environmental risk factors, individual, genetic, family-related, behavioural and lifestyle-related risk factors should also be taken into consideration, as they have a major impact on certain pathologies such as allergic rhinitis and asthma, especially in childhood;

The Italian Study on Asthma in Young Adults (Isaya), a multicentre survey carried out between 1998 and 2000 in nine Italian cities and on 3,000 people between the ages of 20 and 44, highlighted the correlation of the pathology with urban situations with high levels of pollution;

In Italy, it is estimated that every year around ten million people suffer from respiratory allergies due to exposure to allergens from pollen, mould, mites and pets and it is calculated that around 15-20 percent of the Italian population suffers from allergies, a growing phenomenon, especially among young people and women;

The direct costs of asthma, resulting from the use of drugs and health services, represent approximately 1-2% of health expenditure, while the indirect costs (for school absenteeism and reduction of parents' working days due to childcare), in the most serious cases, constitute over 50% of the overall costs, reaching an impact, in economic terms, greater than diseases such as tuberculosis and HIV infection combined;

In the face of a significant epidemiological situation, allergy assistance appears to be significantly reduced at national and regional level and allergic diseases are often not fully considered due to their clinical severity and implications on the quality of life of people, both in developmental age and in adulthood;

Equal access to the use of the most advanced therapies for the treatment of respiratory allergies is not always guaranteed, including desensitization therapies and NPP ("Named Patient Products") regulated by art. 5 of Law no. 94/1998, in line with the principles of therapeutic appropriateness, sustainability for the national health system and equity of access to care in all regions.

This Manifesto is an incentive to protect the rights and access to care for persons with respiratory allergies and to strengthen and rationalize assistance by promoting the growth of large specialist facilities in constant and dynamic connection with the territory.

METHODOLOGICAL NOTE

Public health manifestos are essential tools for communicating important information on disease prevention, health promotion and the management of health emergencies. Their effectiveness depends on how the information is presented, on the clarity of the message and on the visual appeal of the manifesto.

Thanks to the methodological support of BHAVE company for the drafting of the MANIFESTO OF THE RIGHTS AND DUTIES OF THE PERSONS WITH RESPIRATORY ALLERGIES, the following operational path was followed:

1 The first step was to draft a basic text based on international benchmarking on the right to health, on insights provided by participants in the creation of the manifesto and on desk research and analysis on the topic of respiratory allergies.

2 The second step was to receive a review/integration by patient associations and civic representative organizations.

3 The third step involved the review/integration of the text by the Technical-Scientific Committee.

4 The fourth step was based on the verification by qualified external referees of the elements relating to the right to care and health. The referees' task was to verify that what is mentioned in the manifesto is in line with the principle of the right to health as expressed in institutional documents.

5 The fifth step involved the signing and presentation of the manifesto.

SIGNATORIES

PARLIAMENTARY INTERGROUP ON RESPIRATORY ALLERGIES

Association of Italian Allergists of the Territory and Hospital (AAIITO)

"Liberi dall'Asma", from Allergic, Atopic, Respiratory and Rare Diseases adhering to FederASMA and ALLERGIES Italian Patients Federation Odv Association (ALAMA-APS)

"Respiriamo Insieme" Association

Cities+

Cittadinanzattiva

European Academy of Allergy and Clinical Immunology (EAACI)

Federsanità

Health City Institute

Italian Society of Allergology, Asthma and Clinical Immunology (SIAIAC)

Italian Society of Pediatric Allergology and Immunology (SIAIP)

Institute of Translational Pharmacology of the CNR (SIMRI)

Italian Society of General Medicine (SIMG)

Italian Society of Paediatrics (SIP)

Planetary Health Inner Circle

Let's breathe together – TN.
Free from Asthma – TN.
Active Citizenship Association – TN.
Confederation that since 1995 has associated the Local Health Authorities, Hospitals and Scientific Institutes for Hospitalization and Treatment together with the representatives of the Municipalities associated with the national associations of Italian municipalities – TN.

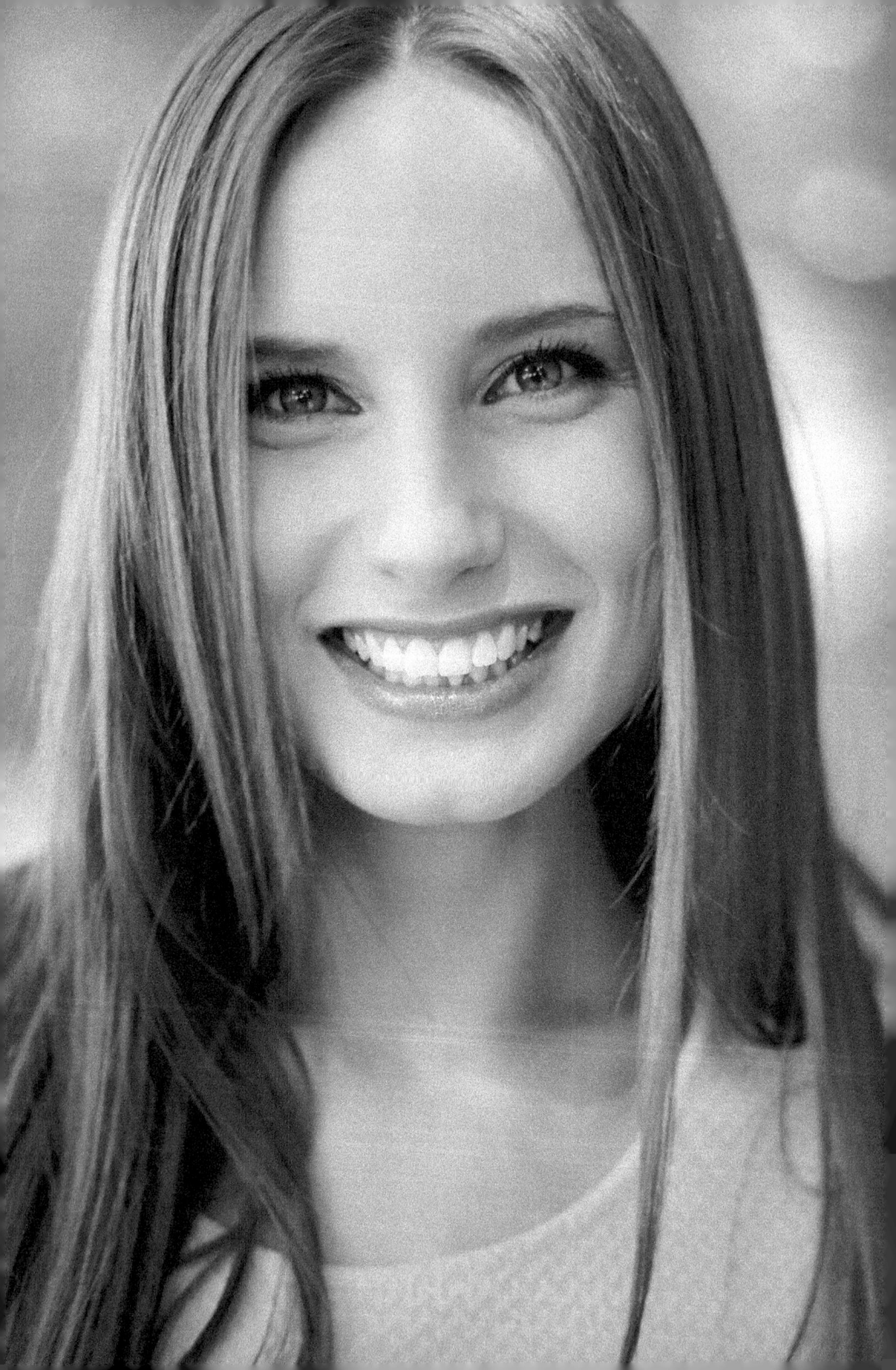

TABLE OF CONTENTS

1. **Rights of the person with respiratory allergies**

2. **Expectations and responsibilities of the person with respiratory allergies and their family members**

3. **Responsible associationism**

4. **Prevention of respiratory allergies**

5. **Remission and control of respiratory allergies**

6. **Commitment to research**

7. **Lifelong education of the person with respiratory allergies**

8. **Communication between doctor and patient with respiratory allergies**

9. **Respiratory allergies in developmental age**

10. **Respiratory allergies in the frail elderly**

11. **Immigration and respiratory allergies**

12. **Territory and respiratory allergies**

The Guideline Act regarding the methods of participation in the decision-making processes of the Ministry of Health by side of Associations or Organizations of citizens and patients involved in health issues, the European Charter of Patients' Rights of Cittadinanzattiva APS, promoted by ACN - European network of Cittadinanzattiva, and the Charter of Rights of the Asthmatic and Allergic Citizen of Federasma and Allergie Odv - Italian Patient Federation, are integral parts of this Manifesto.

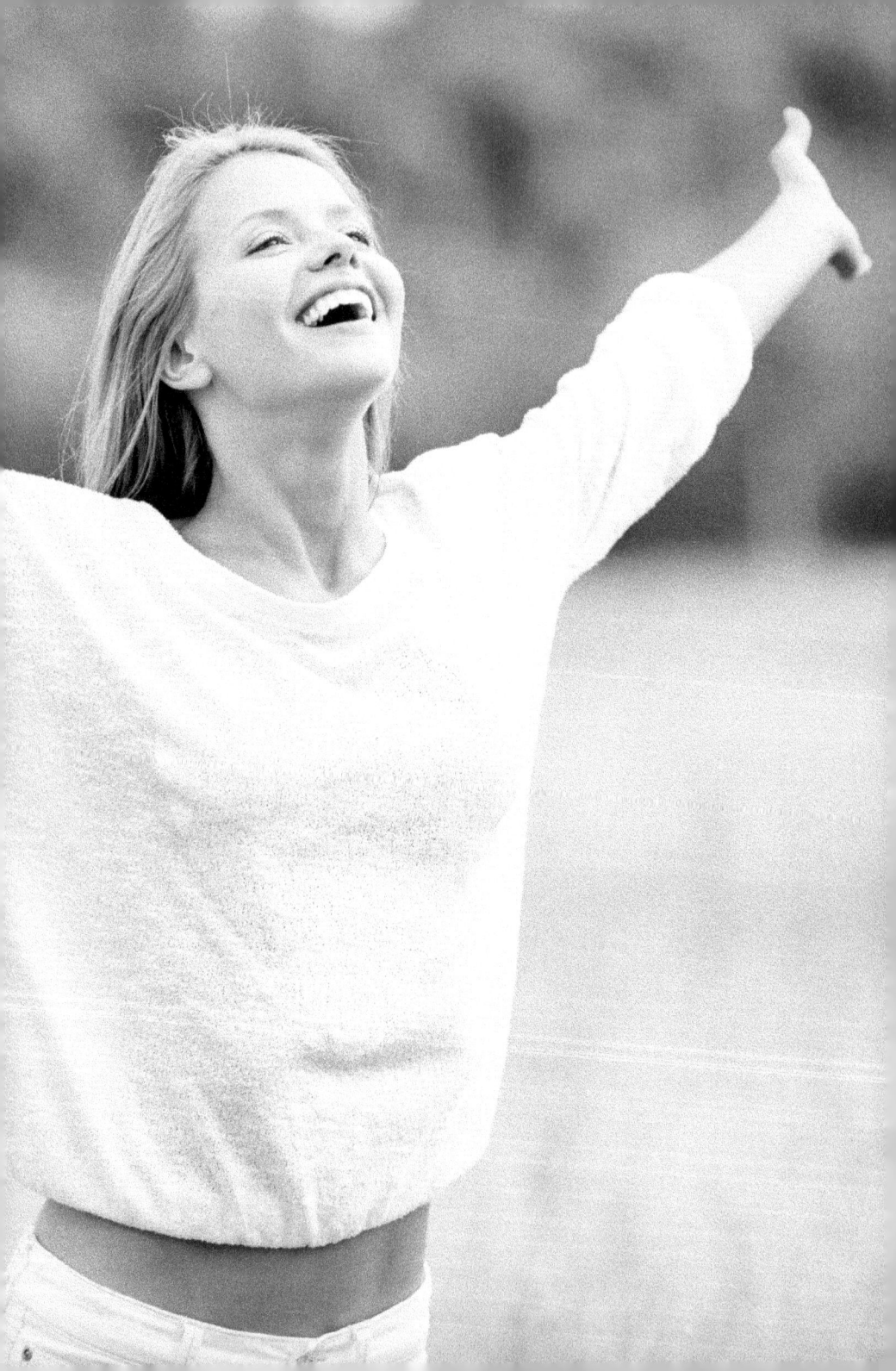

SECTION 1
RIGHTS OF THE PERSON WITH RESPIRATORY ALLERGIES

The rights of those who have respiratory allergies are the same human and social rights as people without respiratory allergies.
The rights include, among others, equal access to information, prevention, therapeutic education, treatment of respiratory allergies and diagnosis and treatment of complications.
The health service must guarantee the person with respiratory allergies access to appropriate diagnostic and therapeutic methods, uniformly throughout the national territory.
The right of people with respiratory allergies to live a social, educational and working life equal to people without respiratory allergies must be considered as an objective of governmental actions.

1. **Affirming** that having respiratory allergies does not preclude the possibility of pursuing (successfully) personal, family, work, sports, school and social goals.

2. **Increasing** awareness of the social impact of respiratory allergies in school, at work, in places where sports are practiced, in health facilities and generally in the whole society in order to avoid discrimination and personal and professional preclusions.

3. **Supporting** the person with respiratory allergies and their family members in overcoming obstacles, prejudices and mistrust through the use of information, training, educational and social tools, together with the empowerment and active participation of institutions, the social-health system, scientific and patient associations, volunteering and civic organizations of people with respiratory allergies.

4. **Ensuring that** people with respiratory allergies have uniform access to the health service throughout the country, in order to promote the best quality of care and life, prevention and treatment of complications with equity.

5. **Educating** social and health workers, teachers and sports instructors, and raise awareness among colleagues on how to prevent, recognize and treat any situations that require urgent intervention.

6. **Promoting** in all regions the guarantee of an early diagnosis of respiratory allergies for all subjects at risk.

7. **Establishing** in all regions, a panel of experts that facilitates interaction and exchange between the different subjects and systems (associations, health service, school system, sports and work systems), in order to handle any requests and applications simply and correctly

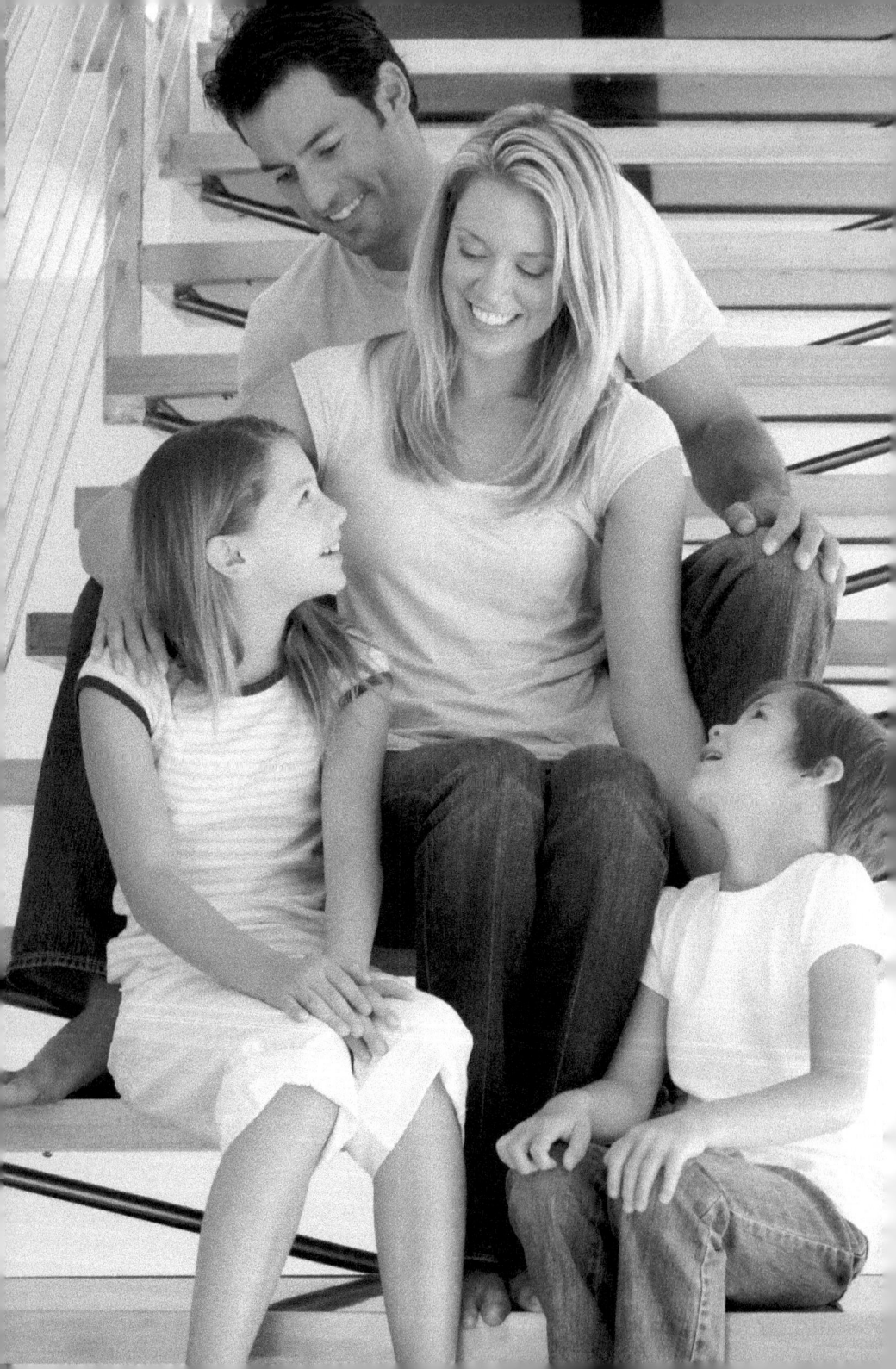

SECTION 2
EXPECTATIONS AND RESPONSIBILITIES OF THE PERSON WITH RESPIRATORY ALLERGIES AND THEIR FAMILY MEMBERS

The person with respiratory allergies and/or their family members are not always aware of the healthcare path and the goals of long-term pharmacological, nutritional and behavioural treatment, as defined by current care guidelines.
The person with respiratory allergies and their family members may mistakenly believe that the situation is "under control" due to the lack of symptoms and therefore decide to suspend the appropriate therapies or modify them inappropriately.
The person with respiratory allergies and their family members must receive correct information on the causes of deficiency, on the risk factors that cause the onset and persistence of respiratory allergies and on the development of complications, so that they are aware of the importance of contrasting them and of leading a healthy lifestyle, in line with their possibilities and needs.

It is therefore necessary to:

1. **Educate** the person with respiratory allergies and their family members so that they can fulfil their life aspirations.

2. **Help** families manage respiratory allergies by providing ongoing training and information, tools and services that take into account the needs of individuals..

3. **Encourage** gli operatori sanitari (specialisti, medici di base, pediatri di famiglia, infermieri, psicologi, ecc..) ad ascoltare attivamente e per un tempo congruo la persona con allergie respiratorie e i familiari per conoscerne i bisogni, le aspirazioni e le aspettative.

4. **Ensure** that healthcare professionals explain the therapeutic objectives in detail, always checking for understanding, and recommend personalized and shared treatment plans (prescribed in both written and oral form) for routine treatment and for any emergency situations.

5. **Invite** all social and health workers to take care of the psychological and social aspects of the person with respiratory allergies and their family members.

6. **Contact** therapy, based on certified diagnostic tests, and to plan scheduled control and follow-up paths.

7. **Ask** persons with respiratory allergies to respect the correct observance to the prescribed therapies, the methods of monitoring respiratory allergies, the lifestyle indications provided by health workers, with the aim of achieving the planned therapeutic objectives in compliance with the resources made available by the health service.

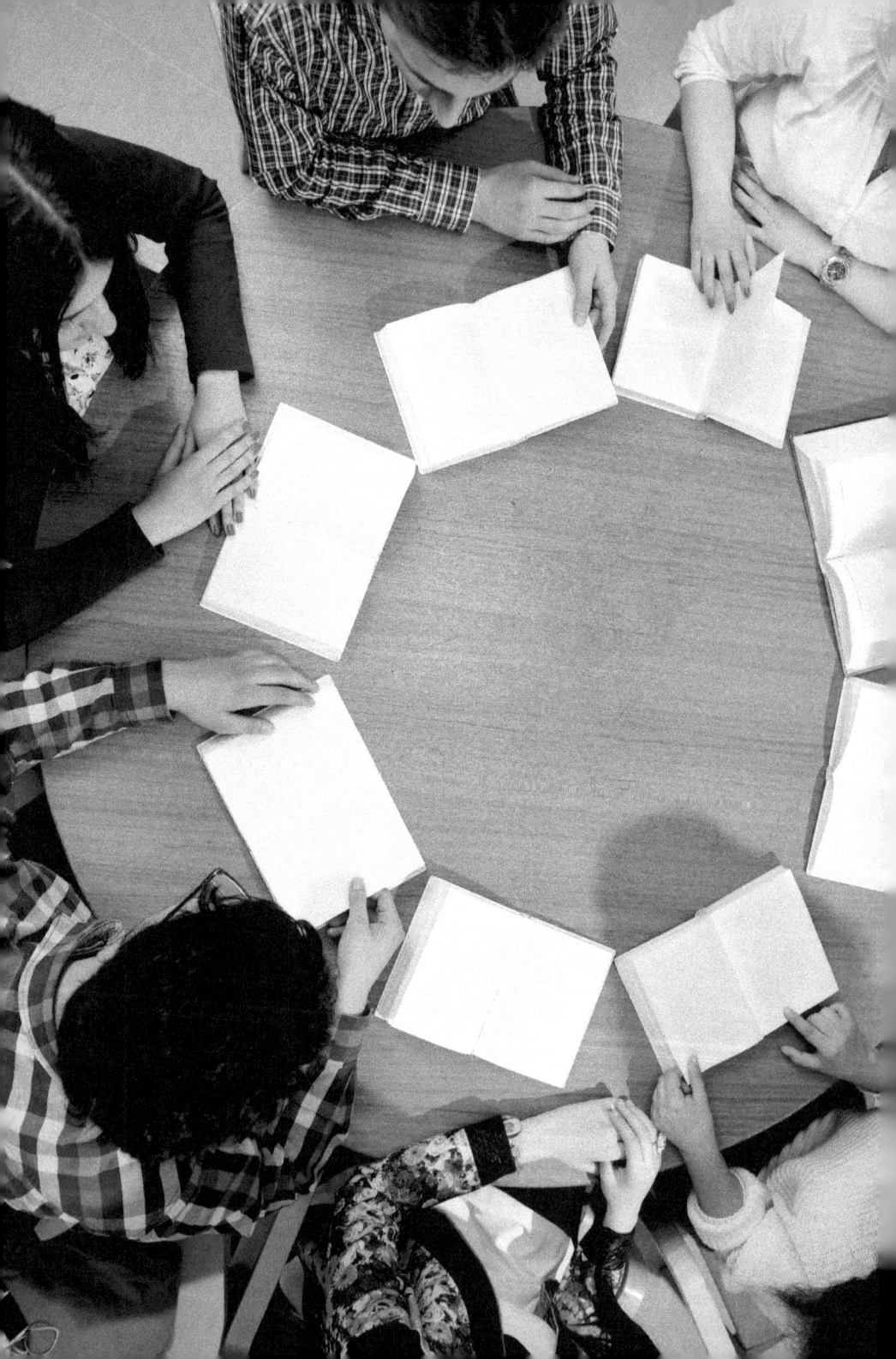

SECTION 3
RESPONSIBLE ASSOCIATIONISM

There are effective preventive measures that can be implemented on the general population to reduce the onset of respiratory allergies by containing their enormous personal and social impact.
For this purpose, a close collaboration is needed between institutions and patient associations, volunteering and civic organizations of persons with respiratory allergies and their families, and scientific societies.
Systematic and ongoing communication activities can promote the prevention and early diagnosis of respiratory allergies, allowing for timely treatment and the reduction of all its consequences.

It is therefore necessary to:

1. **Request** local and national institutions to implement effective strategies for the prevention of respiratory allergies.

2. **Inform** the population that the onset of respiratory allergies can be reduced in people at risk (adults and children) by adopting, where possible, existing suitable therapeutic strategies aimed at the remission of allergies and the prevention of asthma in children.

3. **Convince** institutions to allocate adequate resources for the prevention, early diagnosis and therapeutic strategies of respiratory allergies, and where possible, to avoid or reduce exposure to allergens through continuous and coordinated communication with scientific associations, patient associations, volunteering and civic organizations.

4. **Request** that the competent bodies authorize only in vivo and in vitro diagnostic tests, whose methods must be supported by adequate scientific evidence.

5. **Direct** the institutions to implement allergy clinics and specialist reference centres, equally distributed throughout the country to which the patient can turn in order not to fall into the networks of non-specialized personnel.

6. **Consider** the family, school, work- and recreational places as the privileged places for the development of adequate knowledge of respiratory allergies and education for a correct lifestyle.

7. **Implement** information and health education programs at schools, sports associations, residential centres for the elderly and in general in all living and working environments by involving health institutions, multidisciplinary groups and patient associations, volunteering and civic organizations of people to inform how the correct management of prevention measures and adherence to appropriate therapies allows a lifestyle free from constraints and conditioning.

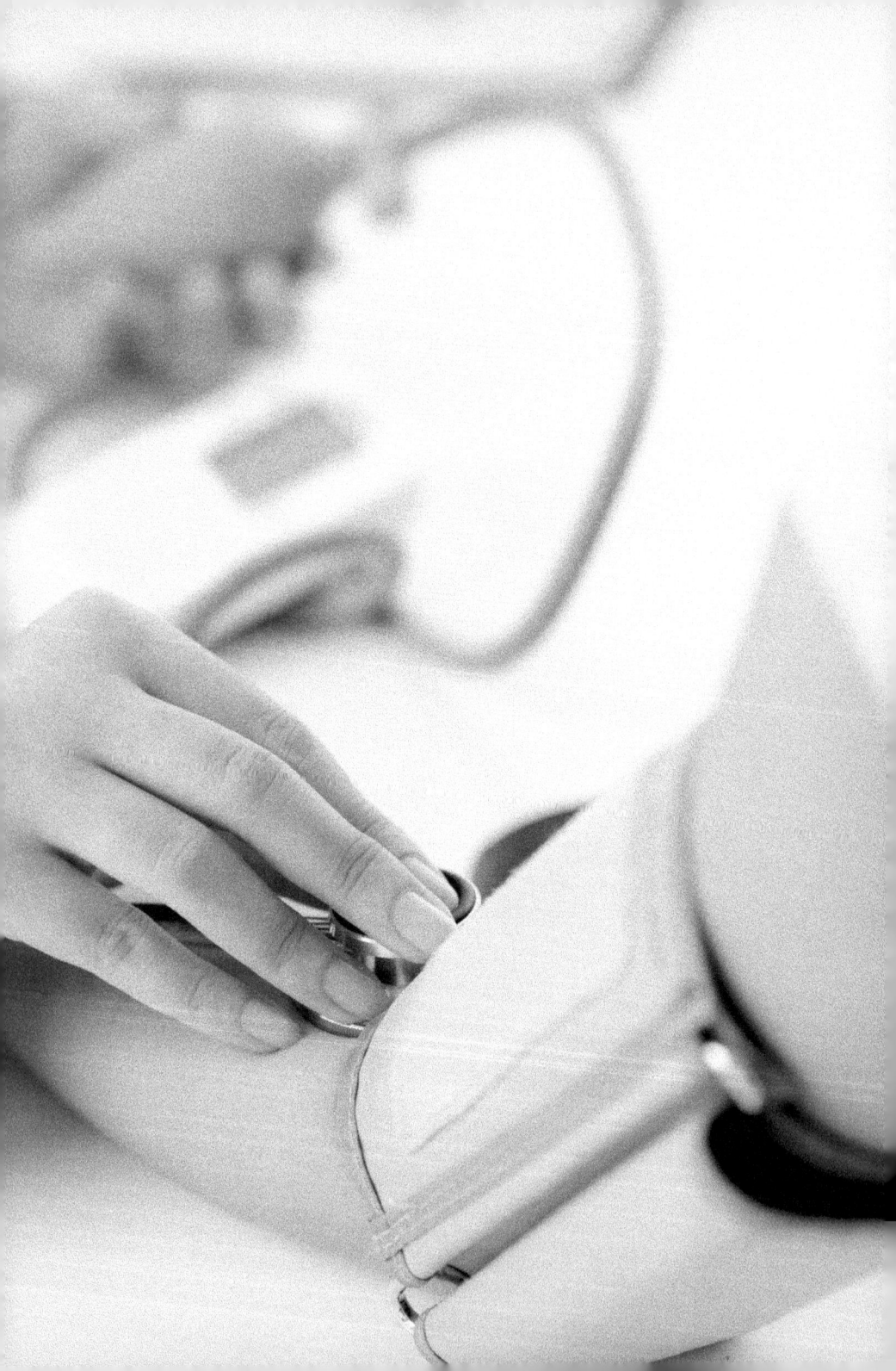

SECTION 4
PREVENTION OF RESPIRATORY ALLERGIES

There are effective preventive measures that can be implemented on the general population to reduce the onset of respiratory allergies by containing their enormous personal and social impact.
For this purpose, a close collaboration is needed between institutions and patient associations, volunteering and civic organizations of persons with respiratory allergies and their families, and scientific societies.
Systematic and ongoing communication activities can promote the prevention and early diagnosis of respiratory allergies, allowing for timely treatment and the reduction of all its consequences.

It is therefore necessary to:

1. **Request** local and national institutions to implement effective strategies for the prevention of respiratory allergies.

2. **Inform** the population that the onset of respiratory allergies can be reduced in people at risk (adults and children) by adopting, where possible, existing suitable therapeutic strategies aimed at the remission of allergies and the prevention of asthma in children.

3. **Convince** institutions to allocate adequate resources for the prevention, early diagnosis and therapeutic strategies of respiratory allergies, and where possible, to avoid or reduce exposure to allergens through continuous and coordinated communication with scientific associations, patient associations, volunteering and civic organizations.

4. **Request** that the competent bodies authorize only in vivo and in vitro diagnostic tests, whose methods must be supported by adequate scientific evidence.

5. **Direct** the institutions to implement allergy clinics and specialist reference centres, equally distributed throughout the country to which the patient can turn in order not to fall into the networks of non-specialized personnel.

6. **Consider** the family, school, work- and recreational places as the privileged places for the development of adequate knowledge of respiratory allergies and education for a correct lifestyle.

7. **Implement** information and health education programs at schools, sports associations, residential centres for the elderly and in general in all living and working environments by involving health institutions, multidisciplinary groups and patient associations, volunteering and civic organizations of people to inform how the correct management of prevention measures and adherence to appropriate therapies allows a lifestyle free from constraints and conditioning.

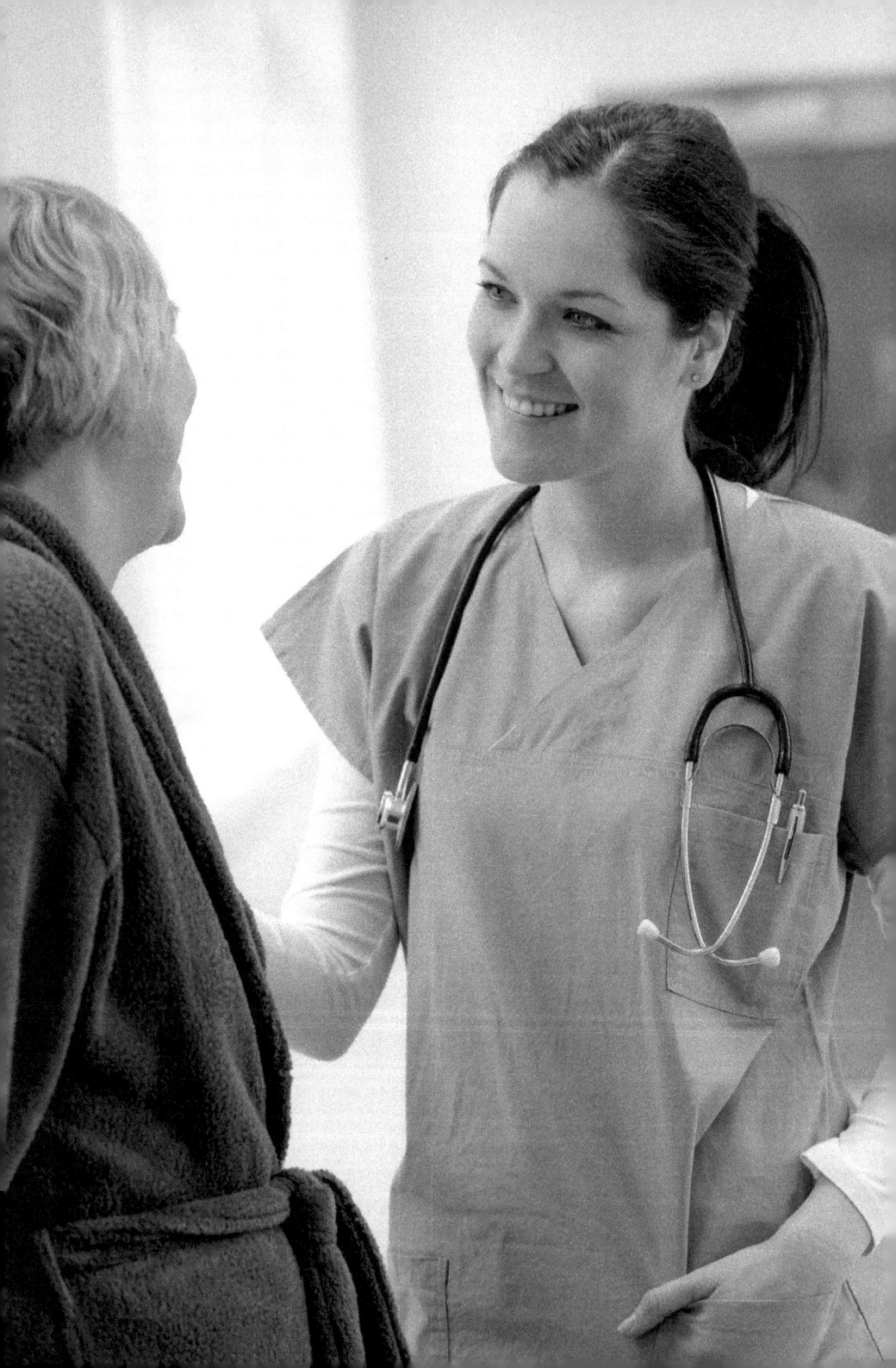

SECTION 5
REMISSION AND CONTROL OF RESPIRATORY ALLERGIES

The person with respiratory allergies must be aware that theirs is a chronic condition, which can either be asymptomatic or with symptoms of varying severity and must be able to manage their own treatment. A correct management of their respiratory allergies allows them to have a school, work, emotional, sports and relational life like that of a person without respiratory allergies. The therapeutic goal is the remission of respiratory allergies to ensure that the patient has control of the symptoms or even no symptoms in the absence of a cortisone-based therapy.

It is therefore necessary to:

1. Increase the knowledge of the appropriate therapies for different clinical conditions in the person with a respiratory allergy and their family members, therapies selected according to the needs and capabilities of the subject, and also of the side effects of some therapies used.

2. Ensure qualified specialist assistance in situations of hospitalization in specialist departments and in order to also guarantee a correct distribution of resources, in territories with an adequate population size, creating or indicating Allergology and Clinical Immunology departments as reference hubs.

3. Facilitate the bureaucratic process and prescription methods to ensure at the national level a homogeneous access to all existing therapies, whether characteristic for the management in the acute phases, or, even more importantly, to therapies that change the natural history of the disease, determining its remission and the related administration tools.

4. Promote appropriate therapeutic programs to encourage a better implementation of clinical protocols so that the care of the person with respiratory allergies also takes place with a view to sustainability of the health service.

5. Inform the person with respiratory allergy and their family members of the possibility of obtaining symptomatic or clinical remission of the disease through a correct treatment, in the absence of a systemic steroid therapy.

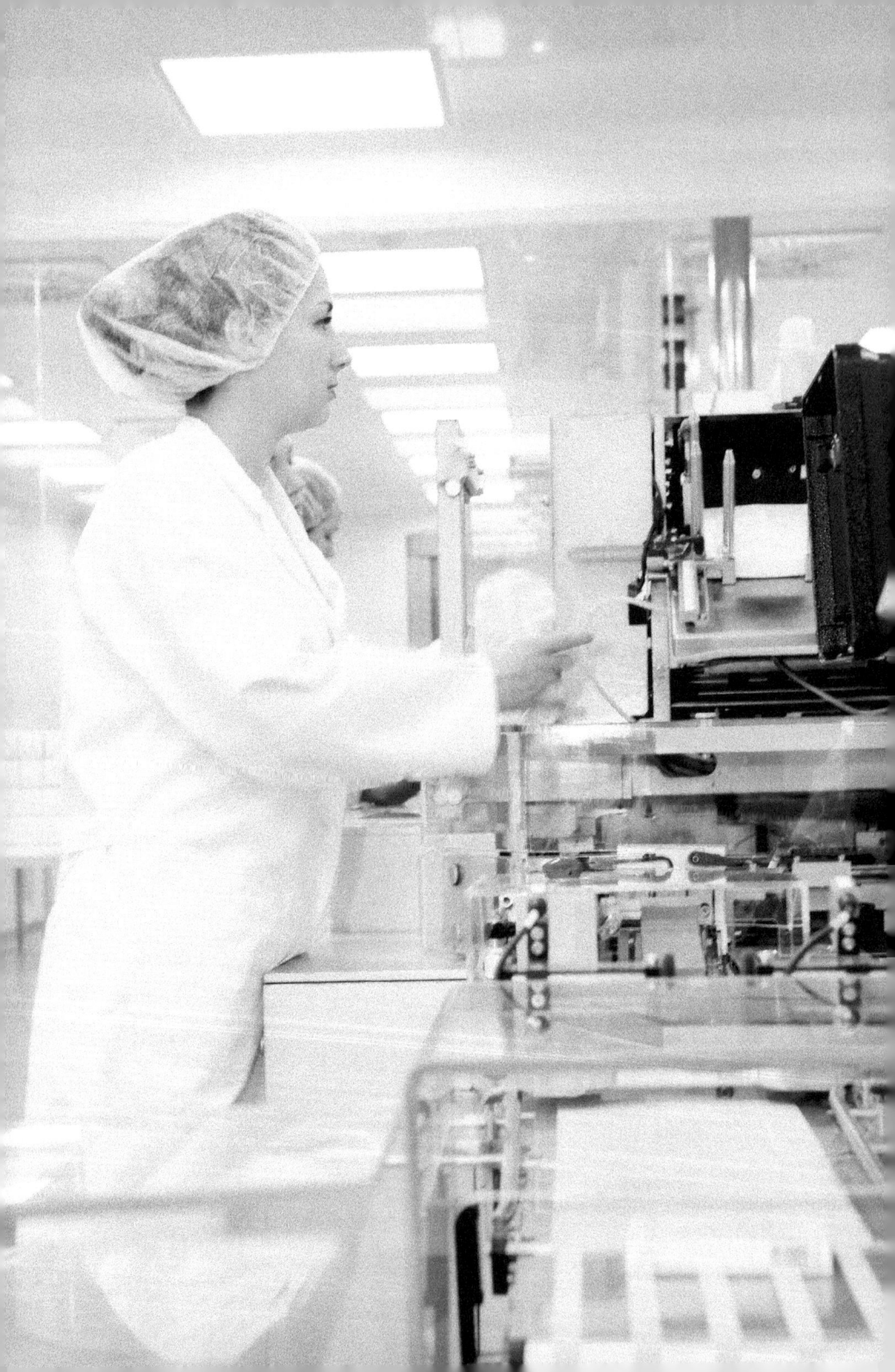

SECTION 6
COMMITMENT TO RESEARCH

Investing in research by side of universities, health institutions, industry, public bodies and scientific societies is a fundamental factor in understanding, preventing and managing respiratory allergies. It is important that research responds to the real needs of persons with respiratory allergies and gets strengthened in the fields of epidemiology, education and technological innovation.

Thanks to the progress in knowledge of respiratory allergies and their treatment, it will be possible to improve the quality of life and prevent the onset of complications, reducing the costs related to the use of symptomatic drugs.

It is therefore necessary to:

1. **Promote** the collaboration between research institutions and patient associations, volunteering and civic organizations of people with respiratory allergies and their families in order to endorse a better understanding of the real needs of patients with respiratory allergies and consequently direct the available resources.

2. **Increase** the resources available for investments in scientific, basic, clinical and epidemiological research, innovation and training.

3. **Promote** studies that aim at achieving a synergy between the therapy that determines the natural history of the disease leading to remission and the sustainability of the National Health System.

4. **Invest** in research and in the application of methodologies and means of communication that allow for the effective spread of thorough information relating to scientific innovations on prevention and integrated management of respiratory allergies and that can promote a correct social representation of the person with respiratory allergies.

5. **Invest** in aerobiological research on the processes of emission and diffusion of allergenic pollens and fungal spores in the atmosphere, taking into consideration the biodiversity of plant species, in particular, in urban environments also in relation to the effects of climate change.

6. **Promote** studies on the interaction between allergenic pollens and air pollution, on the increase in the release of antigens with modified allergenicity and on the greater reactivity of the respiratory tract to inhaled pollen allergens, induced by poor air quality in urban environments.

7. **Develop** a collaborative platform for sharing and integrating the data present in the National Health System databases relating to respiratory allergies, so as to be able to generate a corpus of shared and accessible information for everyone that, by employing technologies such as AI, can go beyond the descriptive analysis but can be of assistance for predictive and prescriptive models.

8. **Promote** the establishment of monitoring registers in order to have a constantly current and evolving picture of Respiratory Allergies throughout the National territory.

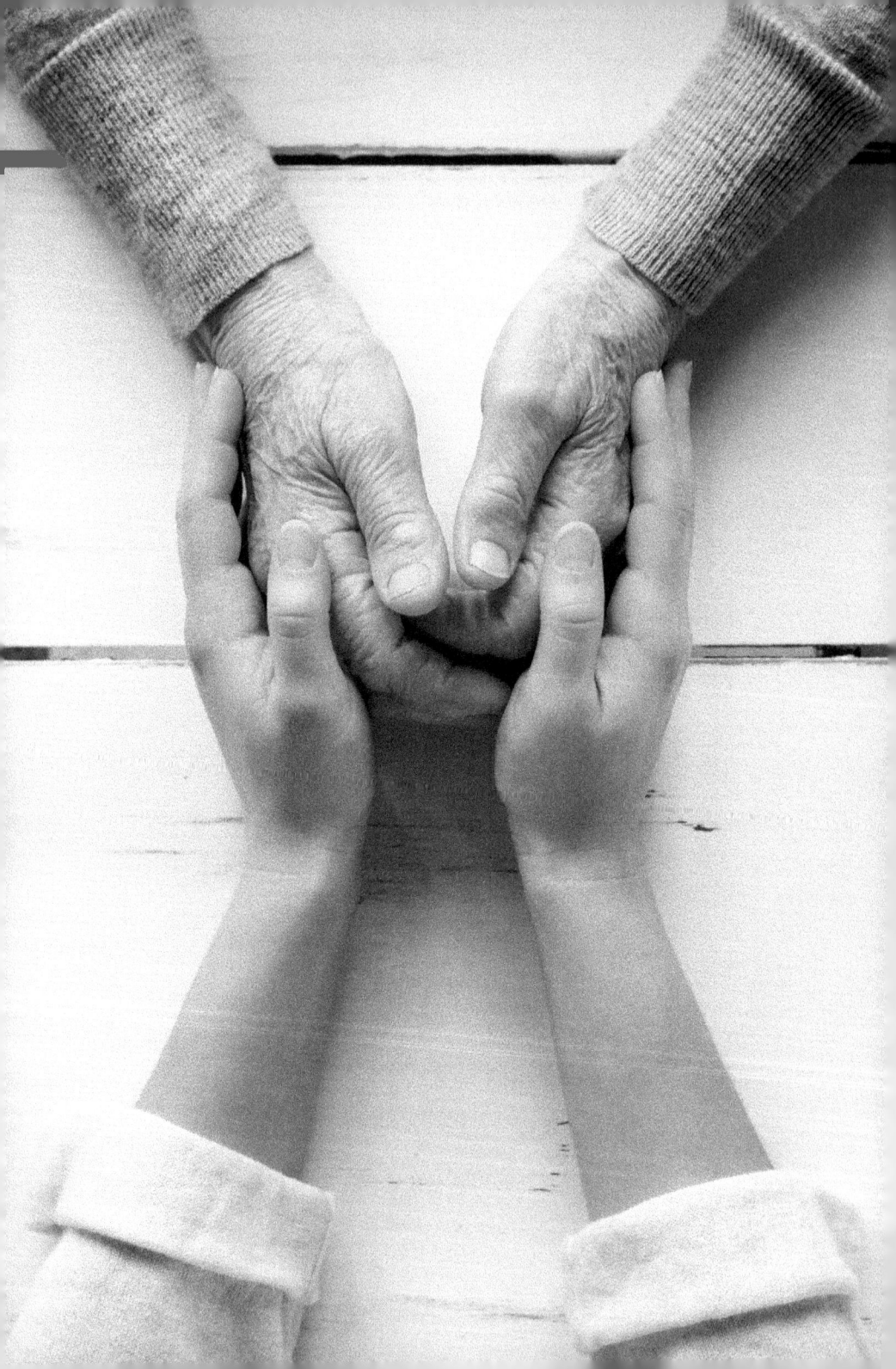

SECTION 7
LIFELONG EDUCATION OF THE PERSON WITH RESPIRATORY ALLERGIES

Lifelong education of the person with respiratory allergies, their family members and the social-relational context is an indispensable tool for achieving full autonomy in the daily management of respiratory allergies and for preventing and recognizing any complications.
It is important to recognize the central role of the educational therapy by providing structured courses.

It is therefore necessary to:

1. Ensure uniformity of access to educational therapy throughout the country.

2. Train healthcare personnel in therapeutic education and volunteering organizations in health education for persons with respiratory allergies and their families, based on their specific clinical and socio-cultural needs.

3. Make use of a multidisciplinary group with specific skills (medical, psychological, nursing, social) useful for removing barriers to a proper handling of respiratory allergies.

4. Share and agree on, after getting some adequate information, the objectives and individualized therapeutic choices in order to facilitate the management of respiratory allergies in daily life.

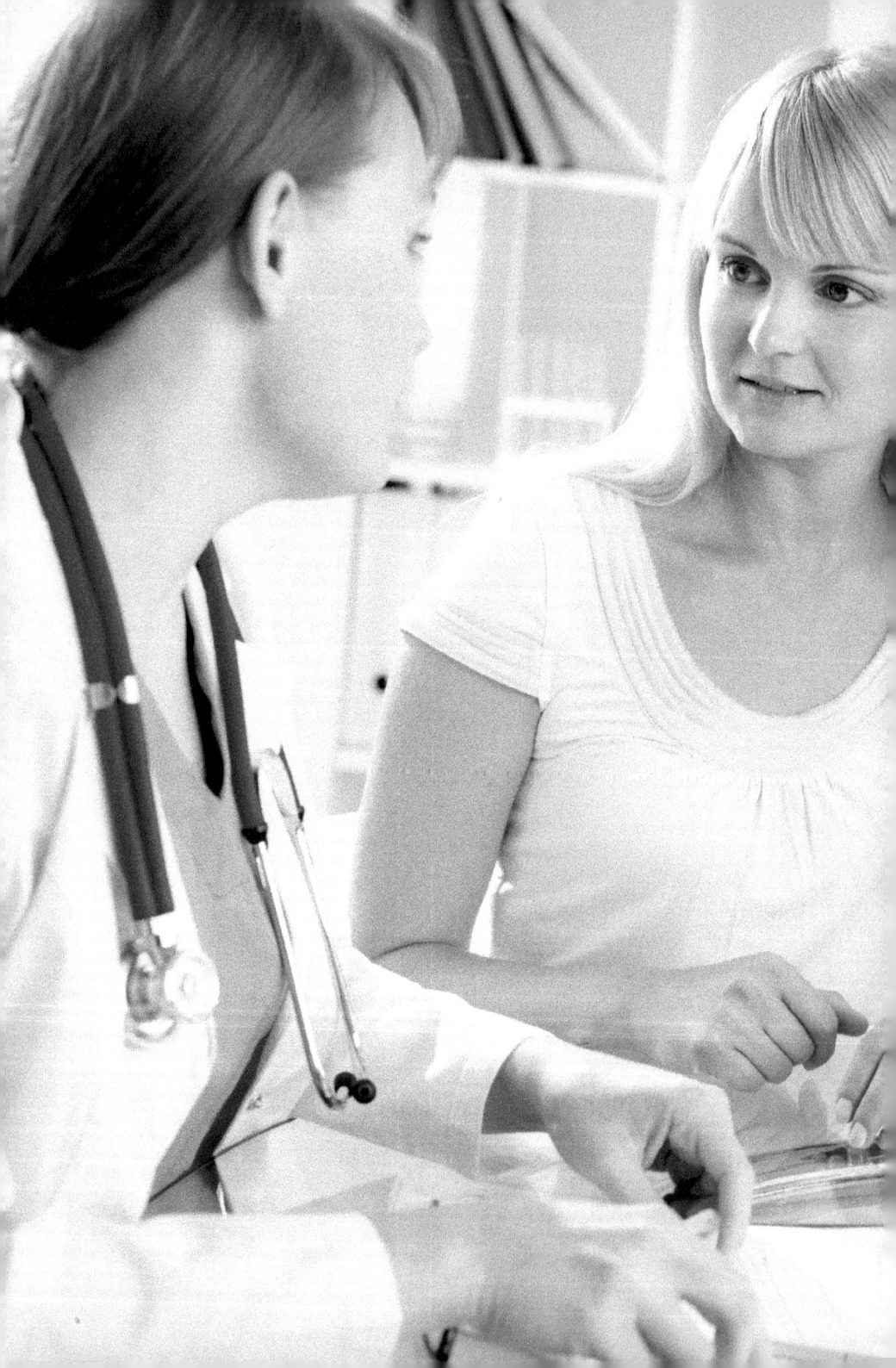

SECTION 8
COMMUNICATION BETWEEN DOCTOR AND PATIENT WITH RESPIRATORY ALLERGIES

To achieve an effective management of respiratory allergies, it is essential that the family physician and the multidisciplinary team of reference know not only the biomedical aspects but also the psychological, relational and social aspects of the person, their perceptions, expectations, needs, obstacles and integrate these elements into the care plan.
To this end, a context must be guaranteed in which the person with respiratory allergies can express their opinions and provide the necessary information about their condition.

It is therefore necessary to:

1. **Ensure** that healthcare professionals establish a real therapeutic alliance with the person with respiratory allergies and their family members that includes active listening, empathetic communication, open dialogue and regular verification not only of the health condition but also of the quality of the service provided.

2. **Invite** healthcare professionals to support the person with respiratory allergies in acquiring full awareness of their condition and their care.

3. **Analyse** individual and family habits and dynamics that may represent risky behaviours.

4. **Facilitate** as much as possible, access and continuity of care even within specialist centres.

5. **Increase** the possibilities and frequency of contact with healthcare professionals also by using modern means of telematic communication, telemedicine and AI (artificial intelligence).

6. **Facilitate** as much as possible, the dialogue between the attending physician/paediatrician and the allergist specialist in order to ensure the application of a common language and strategy.

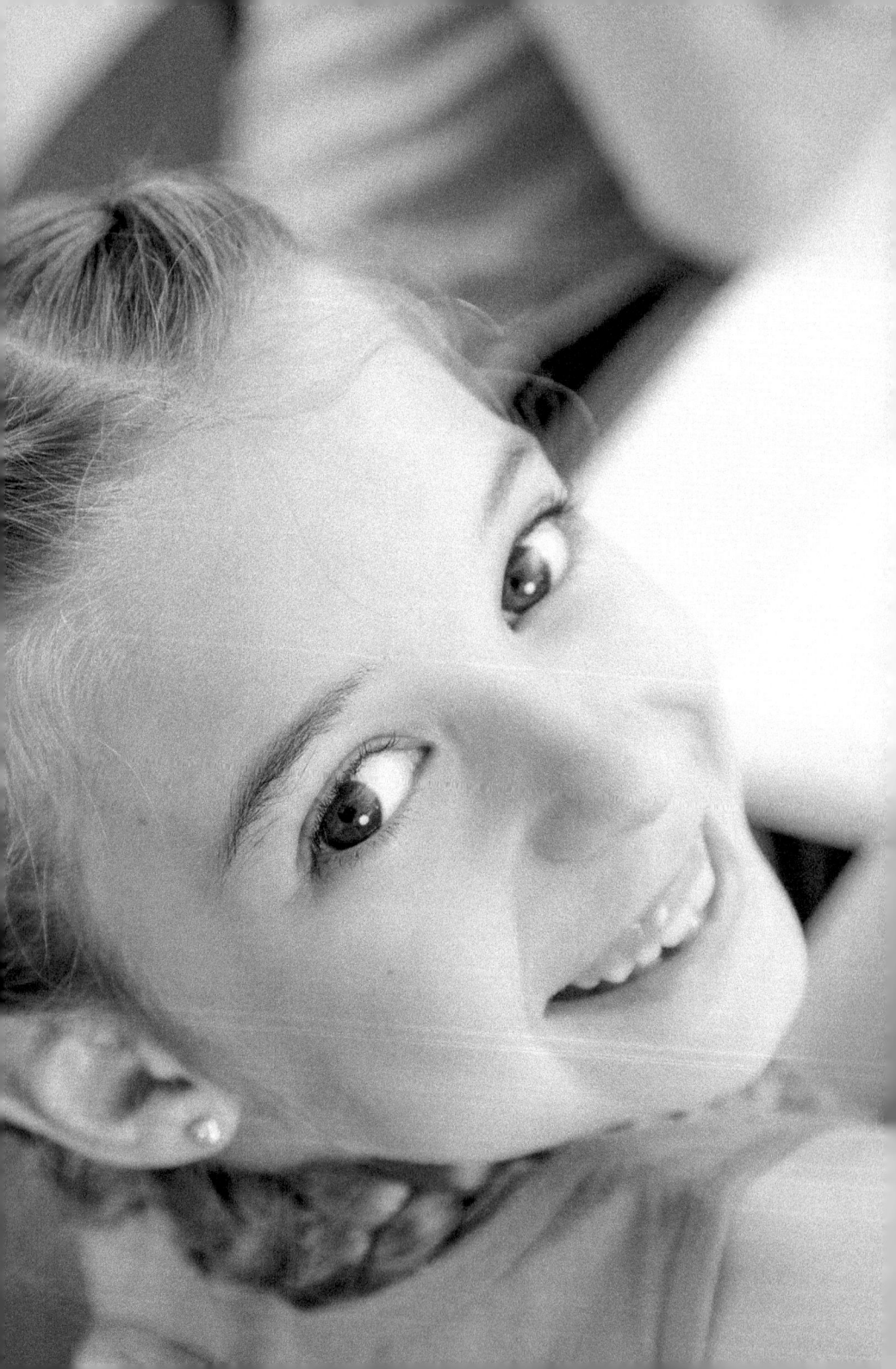

SECTION 9
RESPIRATORY ALLERGIES IN DEVELOPMENTAL AGE

Children and adolescents with respiratory allergies have the right to the most appropriate healthcare services in the paediatric field without any distinction of sex, ethnicity, religion and social condition.
It is a duty to take care of children and adolescents with respiratory allergies, paying particular attention to delicate moments such as schooling and the transition to adult care, which will be managed with specific interventions.

It is therefore necessary to:

1. **Ensure** the best diagnostic process in order to accurately identify the type of respiratory allergies and the therapeutic strategies suitable for the different clinical conditions.
2. **Promote** knowledge of the symptoms for the early diagnosis of respiratory allergies in order to avoid the risks of a late diagnosis.
3. **Ensure** access to the most appropriate treatments, including the innovative ones and the management of comorbidities.
4. **Promote** physical activity, including sports, in the best possible conditions and without any type of limitation.
5. **Support** family members in the management of the child and adolescent with respiratory allergies.
6. **Ensure** that the child and adolescent have a school, sports, relational and social life that meets their needs and desires, to enjoy a good quality of life.
7. **Use** a comprehensible language, appropriate for the age, psycho-physical conditions and culture of the child and family members/guardians.
8. **Ensure** welcoming hospital and outpatient environments, suitable for childhood and adolescence, in which there are dedicated multidisciplinary groups specialized in the treatment of respiratory allergies in this age group and in the assistance of family members/guardians.
9. **Guarantee** that continuity in the assistance of the child and family members/guardians is maintained in Specialized Centres.
10. **Ensure** the ongoing updating of healthcare personnel in order to constantly improve their scientific, technical and communication skills.
11. **Promote** a "network action" in the territory between specialist centres and paediatricians of free choice.
12. **Facilitate** the transition of the adolescent from the paediatric specialist to the adult specialist in order to guarantee a continuity of care; this process must occur gradually, through the sharing of objectives and therapeutic choices involving their referring doctors (Paediatricians of Free Choice, GPs and specialist doctors).

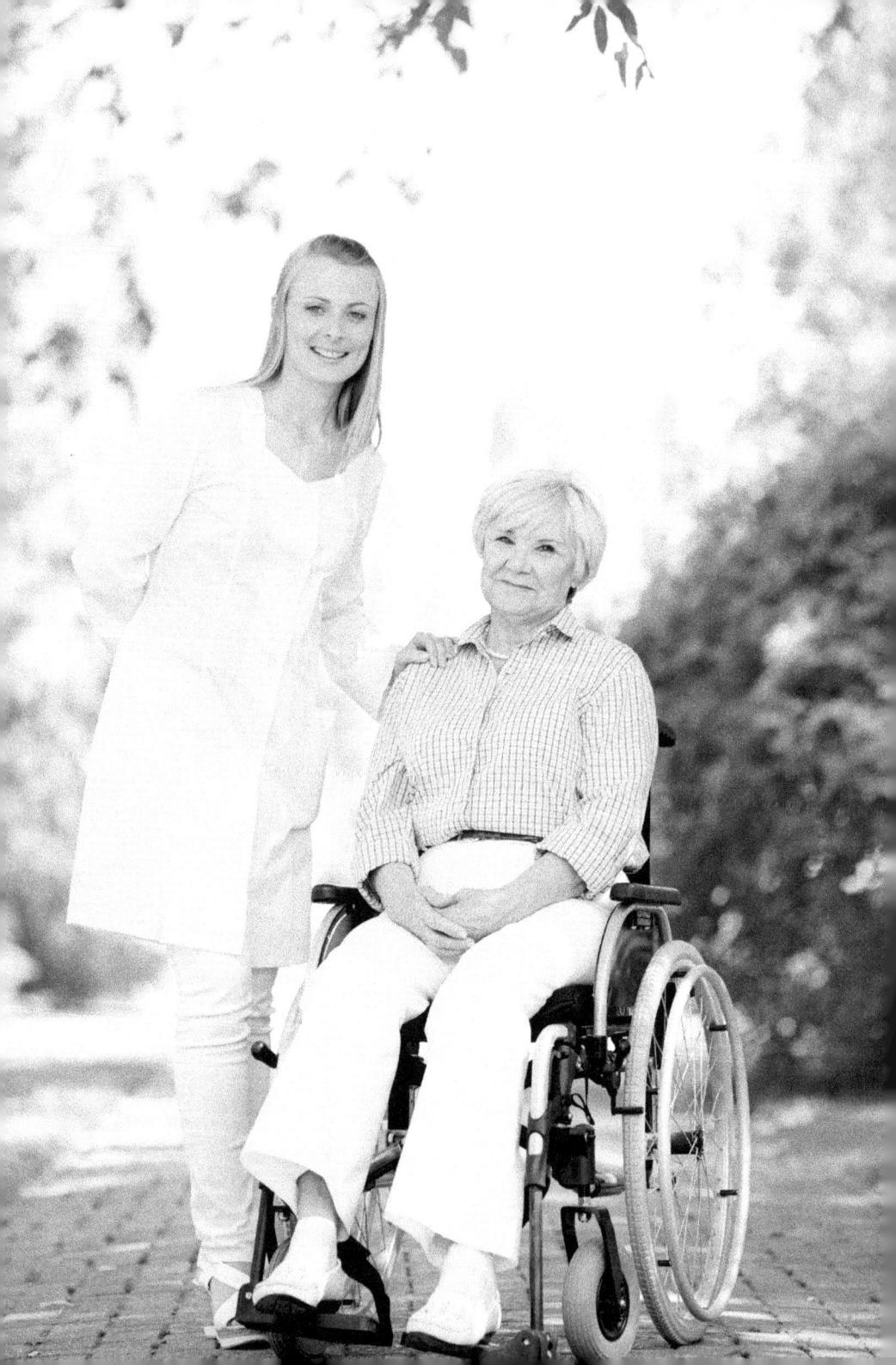

SECTION 10
RESPIRATORY ALLERGIES IN THE FRAIL ELDERLY

The frail elderly with respiratory allergies have the right to the best health services without any social or cultural discrimination, so that they can continue to have an active role in community life. It is necessary to take care of the frail elderly with respiratory allergies, paying particular attention to their general health conditions, cognitive conditions, concomitant pathologies and the context in which they live in order to design personalized and easily applicable therapies, and to educate them about constant home care, if necessary, and the adoption of correct lifestyles.

It is therefore necessary to:

1. Ensure dedicated facilities that take into account the specific needs of the frail elderly with respiratory allergies (rooms with dedicated devices, limited waiting times and sufficient visit times for adequate information and training, by specifically trained healthcare workers).

2. Use a clear and comprehensible written and oral language that is appropriate for the culture and psycho-physical state of the frail elderly with respiratory allergies and their family members/caregivers.

3. Promote home interventions and the role of local territorial facilities in the management of the frail elderly with respiratory allergies so as to guarantee continuity of care by a multifunctional and multiprofessional team.

4. Support families/caregivers with adequate training, which prepares them and makes them autonomous in handling the care of the elderly/frail subject with respiratory allergies who are not self-sufficient, and with suitable support to take care of them also from a psycho-emotional perspective.

5. Promote interventions and actions that favour the maintenance of social and friendly life for elderly people with respiratory allergies for the maintenance of an active life, also through the availability of risk-free spaces/places.

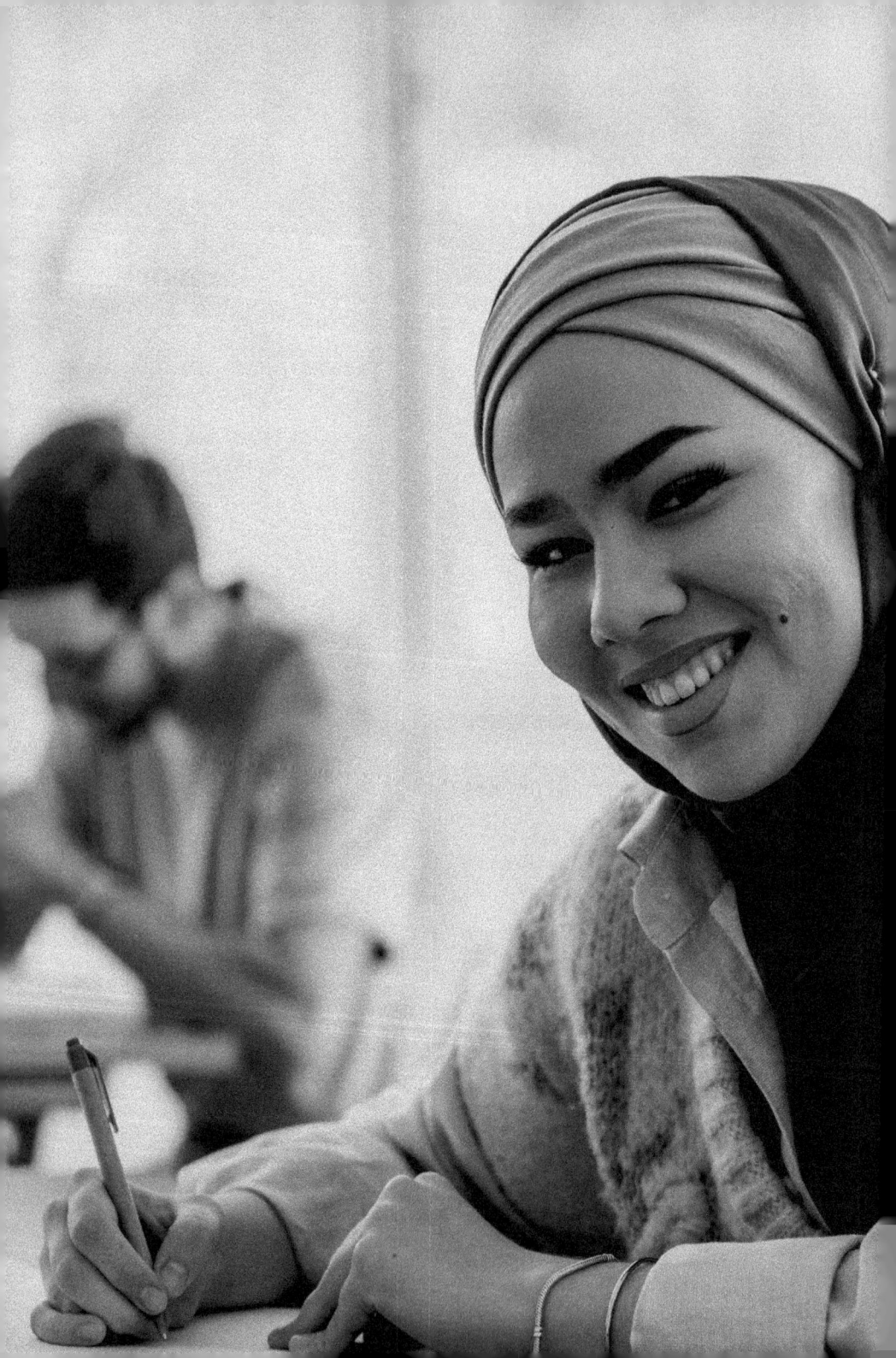

SECTION 11
IMMIGRATION AND RESPIRATORY ALLERGIES

A person with respiratory allergies must not be discriminated against on the base of their language, ethnicity, geographical origin, religion, psycho-physical condition and status.

It is therefore necessary to:

1. **Facilitate** the access to healthcare services throughout the country for immigrants of all ages who suffer from or are at risk of respiratory allergies, with the use of linguistic mediation services.

2. **Adjust** where possible, treatment programs for people with respiratory allergies to the customs dictated by cultural and religious traditions if not in conflict with human rights and therapeutic needs.

3. **Offer** ongoing education courses held by multidisciplinary groups, supported by staff from patient associations, volunteering and civic organizations of people with respiratory allergies and their families who are able to communicate multilingually in all living and working environments.

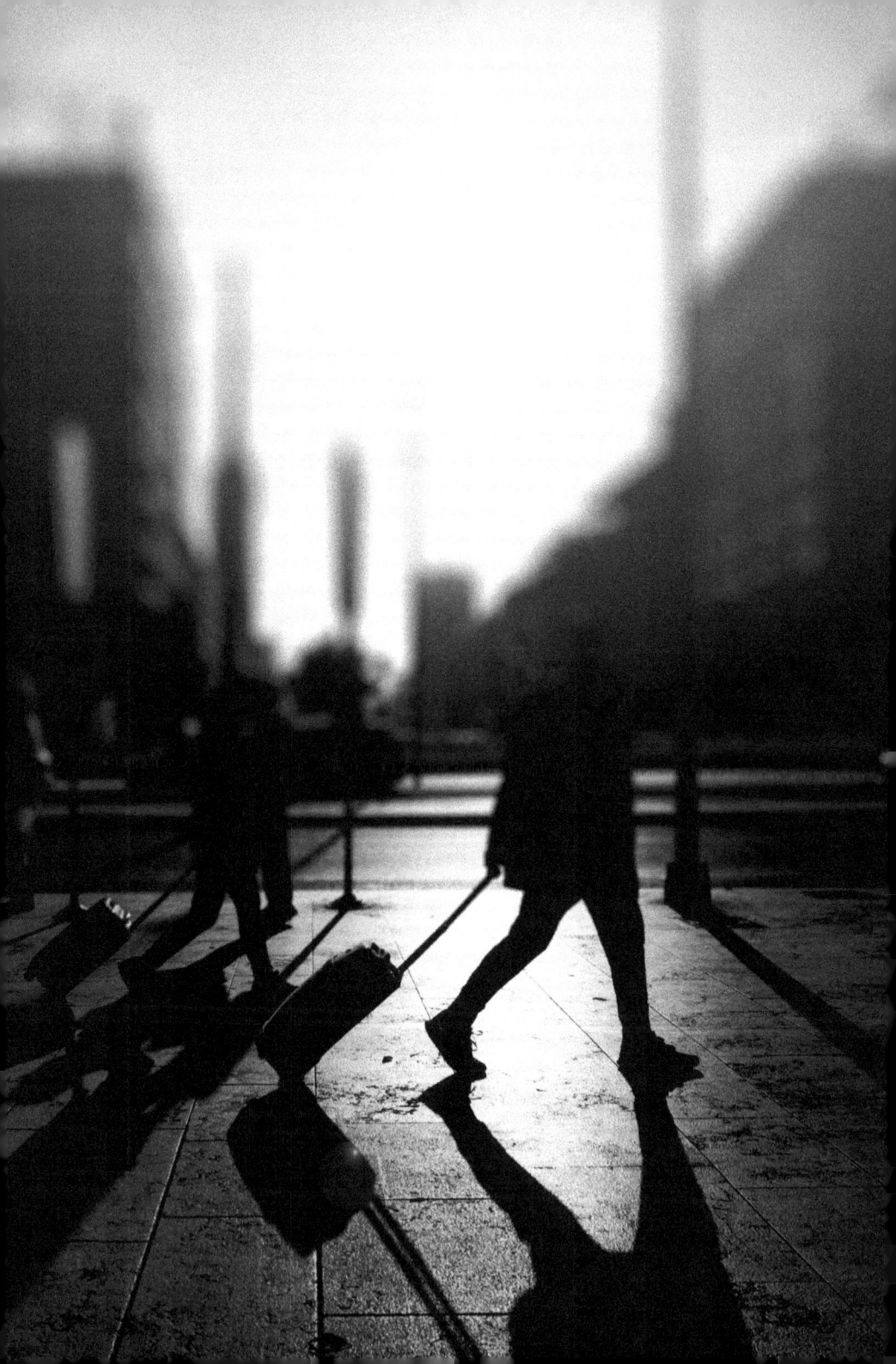

SECTION 12
TERRITORY AND RESPIRATORY ALLERGIES

The analysis and continuous monitoring of respiratory allergy data allow us to identify short, medium and long-term strategies that can determine management changes and help spread the culture of prevention as a tool to reduce the incidence of respiratory allergies on the population and the social and economic costs resulting from the treatment of its complications. At the same time, monitoring the biological component of airborne particulate matter in the atmosphere allows us to produce extremely useful information in the diagnosis, clinic, therapy, research and prevention of respiratory allergic diseases.

Through specific studies carried out at the territorial and national level, it is possible to understand the geographical and cultural characteristics that can determine the onset of respiratory allergies, to increase the socio-political awareness and to raise and standardize treatment standards throughout the country to effectively meet the treatment needs.

It is therefore necessary to:

1. Promote the implementation of a National and Regional Plan for respiratory allergies through specific intervention policies, so as to make the therapeutic-care pathway uniform throughout the national territory, in order to avoid or oppose existing discrepancies.

2. Support local and national observatories on respiratory allergies in their data collection and analysis activity, necessary for understanding all the aspects that cause the onset of respiratory allergies and for evaluating the quality of the care provided.

3. Use the available evidence within public awareness campaigns, shared and jointly promoted by institutions, healthcare and associations.

4. Ensure an integrated healthcare organization that contributes to changing lifestyles, the environment in which we live, related to the risk of respiratory allergies, as well as provide innovative healthcare services in an equitable manner.

5. Promote the aerobiological monitoring of allergenic pollens and fungal spores through measurement sites, arranged in a network, spread throughout the national territory.

6. Activate shared protocols between/with Local Authorities, Institutions, Associations, for the management of public and school green spaces, in order to adopt management and maintenance measures for green spaces with the aim of reducing/mitigating the presence of invasive and allergenic species, with particular reference to residential areas.

MANIFESTO OF THE RIGHTS AND DUTIES OF PERSONS WITH RESPIRATORY ALLERGIES

With the unconditional contribution of

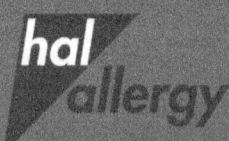

Nella stessa collana

Trasforma le tue idee in un libro — Denise Cumella
Il packaging per il tuo successo — Daniele Barbato e Giuseppe Muollo
Anniversario Aziendale — Cumella, Redana, Jossi e Di Maggio
Visionary HR — Deborah Palma
Processi semplici davvero! — Paolo Balestra
Gli alberi che ascoltano — Mima Muratovic e Martina Osti
Experience: un viaggio nel gusto — Giuseppe Naclerio
Vision is not a choice — Luca Piras e Emanuele D'Arrigo
Sicurezza Operativa — Mario Stigliano
I numeri comandano — Mirco Gasparotto
Intelligenza Patrimoniale — Giovanni Cuniberti
+1 — Jonathan Sitzia
Memorie di un avvocato milanese — Avv. Luciano Di Pardo
Vendere con il sorriso — Achille Carcagnì
Energia da vendere — Alessandro Basilico
La Magia del Biotermocamino — De Luca Rocco
Longevità finanziaria — Filippo Montaina
Mai più schiavi del denaro — Mirko Tessari
Libera la tua luce e volta pagina — Alessandro Comella
Clienti Forever — Giuseppe Foderà
Recruiting Marketing — Michele Andreano
Il Futuro del monouso — Michele e Angelo Raffaele Guadagno
La finanza agevolata nello shipping — Alessandro Pasti
Banking Secrets — Gennaro Baccile e Stefano Cesare Palazzi
10 segreti per vendere il tuo immobile di pregio — Andrea Galli
Fai decollare la tua impresa — Giuseppe D'Errico
L'azienda con i superpoteri — Corrado Malighetti
Cambia la percezione del tuo brand — Riccardo Urso
I soldi son desideri — Ferdinando Scavone
La rivincita dei quattrocchi — Arianna Foscarini
Butta via i fazzoletti — Sabrina De Federicis
Verifica la bontà dei tuoi investimenti — Giuseppe Tocchetti
Viaggio al centro della finanza — Filippo Montaina
Internazionalizza la tua impresa — Igor Pahor
Tu sei un Eroe, Volume I — Francesco Cardone
Brain your sales up, Edizione italiana — Daniele Casuccio

Change Marketing — Marco Daturi
Cibo in rosa — Emiliana Giusti
Ricominciare da zero con il fashion franchising — Eduardo Capobianco
La bussola della digitalizzazione — Alessio Angioli
La Finanziata ideale — Alessandro Trentin
Trova la persona giusta per la tua azienda — Ciro Nicolò Del Sorbo e Imma Santonicola
Spedire a Natale è facile (se sai come farlo) — Cristian Fazi
Non è vero che il nero sfina — Cinzia Catozzi e Lidia Colognola
Il Giro del Mondo in 40 giorni — Massimiliano Loyola
Rivoluzione paid traffic — Marco Sepertino
Turbolenze condominiali — Paolo Cesareo
Basta lamentarsi! — Antonio Guttilla
I codici segreti delle reti vendita — Roberto Giangregorio
Il valore del comfort acustico — Oscar Avian
Imprenditore di pregio — Andrea Galli e Matteo Stella
Liberati dal dolore (on line) — Tiziana Tonelli
Nutriti di energia — Alice Fazi
Imprenditori che cambiano — Michela Canova e Francesca Caputo
Amministra condominî senza rubare — Paolo Traverso
Come vendere di più con YouTube — Paolo Grisendi
Intelligenza aziendale — Paolo Balestra
La video rinascita — Placido Losacco
Innova senza errori — Sebastiano Gadaleta
Più colore al tuo business — Fenix Digital Group
L'amianto non fa male (al portafoglio) — Leonardo Mormandi
Formazione Cinica — Luca Favale
Il piacere di stare bene — Cristina Caputo
Spedire è facile (se sai come farlo) — Cristian Fazi
Metodo Giusti — Emiliana Giusti
Da dipendente a imprenditore — Feliciano Lorenzo di Giovambattista
Personal Trainer Marketing — Corrado Pirovano
Il Signore di Londra — Davide Catalano
Inventa il tuo futuro come ho fatto io — Aldo Corbo
Il tuo infermiere — Gioacchino Costa
Stretto d'Autore — Gaetano Bevacqua
La scomoda verità sui contributi a fondo perduto — Salvatore Reina
Azienda No Problem — Guido Fornari
Vendere Fitness — Luigi Cacciapaglia

Impatto Funnel Marketing — Michele Tampieri e Alessandro Bentivoglio
Impresa Vincente — Francesco Cardone
CEO Second Life — Matteo Fini
Supera quel dannato milione — Carmine Lamberti
L'importante non è vincere ma stravincere — Francesco Giffi
Comunità energetiche — Alessandro Basilico
La mia grande impresa — Massimo Labruna
Igiene e cura per cani e gatti — Pietro Maccarone
Calamite digitali — Antonio Mariggiò
Una vita a tutto gas — Graziella Cianciotto

All cases reported in the text are real.
For privacy reasons, fictitious names have been used.

www.ingramcontent.com/pod-product-compliance
Lightning Source LLC
LaVergne TN
LVHW061046070526
838201LV00074B/5198